The Syringe Driver

The Syringe Driver
Continuous subcutaneous infusions in palliative care

Andrew Dickman
Specialist Principal Pharmacist, Palliative Care Team,
Whiston Hospital, Prescot, Merseyside, UK

Clare Littlewood
Palliative Care Consultant, Whiston Hospital, Prescot,
Merseyside, UK

James Varga
Palliative Care Pharmacist, Pain and Palliative Care
Association, Florida, USA

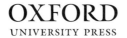

OXFORD
UNIVERSITY PRESS

OXFORD
UNIVERSITY PRESS

Great Clarendon Street, Oxford OX2 6DP

Oxford University Press is a department of the University of Oxford.
It furthers the University's objective of excellence in research, scholarship,
and education by publishing worldwide in

Oxford New York

Auckland Bangkok Buenos Aires Cape Town Chennai Dar es Salaam
Delhi Hong Kong Istanbul Karachi Kolkata Kuala Lumpur Madrid
Melbourne Mexico City Mumbai Nairobi São Paulo Shanghai
Singapore Taipei Tokyo Toronto

and an associated company in Berlin

Oxford is a registered trade mark of Oxford University Press
in the UK and in certain other countries

Published in the United States
by Oxford University Press Inc., New York

© Dickman, Littlewood and Varga, 2002

The moral rights of the author have been asserted

Database right Oxford University Press (maker)

First published 2002

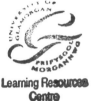

British Library Cataloguing in Publication Data

Data available

Library of Congress Cataloguing in Publication Data

ISBN 0-19-851550 2 (Pbk)

10 9 8 7 6 5 4 3 2 1

Typeset by EXPO Holdings, Malaysia
Printed in Great Britain
on acid-free paper by T. J. International Ltd

Contents

Foreword

Palliative medicine continues to widen its horizons. It is heartening to see the common practice of continuous subcutaneous infusion of medications being used by our colleagues across the world. We hope this new text will provide a useful resource to all, and continue to enhance the multiprofessional approach of the discipline.

Acknowledgements

The authors wish to thank Dr Duke Dickerson and Dr Nathan Cherny; without their initial interest and enthusiasm, this book would not have been published. Thanks are also due to Willowbrook Hospice, Merseyside, UK where all the clinical outcomes were assessed. In addition, the authors would like to thank the reviewers Miss Sharon Dry, Dr Anthony Thompson and Mrs Jackie Williams.

List of Abbreviations

General

CNS	Central nervous system
CSCI	Continuous subcutaneous infusion
CTZ	Chemoreceptor trigger zone
IM	Intramuscular
IV	Intravenous
m/r	Modified release
po	Per os (by mouth)
PVC	Polyvinyl chloride
sc	Subcutaneous
UK	United Kingdom
WHO	World Heath Organization

Medical

D_2	Dopamine type 2 (receptor)
H_1, H_2	Histamine type 1, 2 (receptor)
$5\text{-}HT_1, 5\text{-}HT_2, 5\text{-}HT_3$	5 hydroxytriptamine (serotonin) receptors
μ	opioid (receptor)
κ	Kappa opioid (receptor)
δ	Delta opioid (receptor)
α_2	Alpha type 2 adrenergic (receptor)
M	Muscarinic (receptor)
M3G	Morphine-3-glucuronide
M6G	Morphine-6-glucuronide
NMDA	N-methy-D-aspartate
NSAID(s)	Non-steroidal anti-inflammatory drug(s)

Units

ml	Millilitre(s)
mg	Milligram(s)
h	Hour(s)

Introduction

Palliative care patients often exhibit multiple symptoms that require polypharmacy. Unfortunately, a given patient's condition may deteriorate, such that oral administration is no longer possible. In such circumstances, the syringe driver can be used to ensure continued symptom control.

Situations routinely arise that require combinations of two or three drugs in the same syringe. Occasionally, four or even five drugs may be given this way, although it is important to ensure that the drugs are pharmacologically distinct. It is surprising that evidence for this practice is very difficult to locate.

This book serves as a valuable reference source, providing extensive information pertaining to the use of continuous subcutaneous infusions. The first chapter provides an overview of syringe drivers and continuous subcutaneous infusions. It focuses on the portable devices produced by SIMS Graseby, the MS16A and MS26. The second chapter provides referenced information about drugs that are likely to be encountered, including certain drugs that should only be used by, or on the recommendation of, a palliative care specialist. The third chapter provides information relating to the control of specific symptoms that are often encountered when continuous subcutaneous infusions are required. The fourth and final chapter contains an extensive list of physical stability data relating to drug combinations used for subcutaneous administration.

All information included in this book is correct at the time of writing. With the exceptions of diamorphine and levomepromazine, the subcutaneous infusions of drugs mentioned within this book are outside current UK product licences. Practitioners in other countries are advised to check local information. Whilst every effort has been made to ensure accuracy, responsibility remains with the prescriber. Neither the authors nor publisher can accept responsibility for any errors or omissions that may be made.

Important note

Physical stability data comes from two sources in this book—the laboratory and the clinical setting. Mixtures within this book are termed physically compatible if they remained colourless, clear and free from particular matter over the specified time; additionally, for clinical data, the expected outcome was realised.

References to chemical stability, where available, will be found under each drug section in Chapter 2.

Finally, stability data mentioned here can only serve as an indicator and may not apply to all situations.

Chapter 1

Continuous subcutaneous infusions and syringe drivers

Introducing the syringe driver

A continuous subcutaneous infusion (CSCI) is an extremely useful method of drug administration, particularly suited to palliative care. Although the oral route is preferable, a patient's condition may deteriorate such that it is no longer possible to administer drugs this way. There are a variety of reasons why a syringe driver might be needed, and it is important to dispel the myth that its use means the end of life is approaching. Rectal administration is not always practical and the patient may find it unacceptable. Intravenous injections should be avoided, particularly as CSCIs are less invasive and have been found to be as effective. Intramuscular administration will be painful, especially if the patient is cachectic.

There are currently two types of SIMS Graseby® syringe drivers suitable for use: the MS16A (Fig. 1) and the MS26 (Fig. 2). The MS26 is probably the simplest and safest to use and is therefore recommended in the palliative care setting.

The MS26 has a boost button. The use of this is not recommended for several reasons:

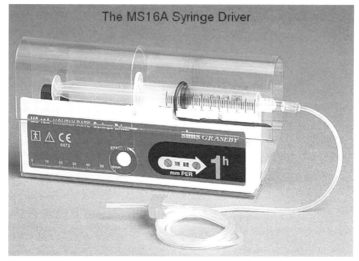

Fig. 1 The MS16A.

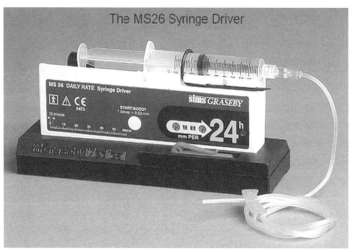

Fig. 2 The MS26.

The differences

The main important difference between the syringe drivers is that the MS26 delivers at a rate set in millimeters per 24 hours, whereas the MS16A delivers at a rate set in millimeters per hour. Note that delivery is based on a length of liquid and not volume.

1 There is no lock-out period. Once the boost button is depressed, the device delivers eight boosts and alarms. The infusion continues. If the button is released and depressed again, up to another eight boosts will be delivered, and so on. Hence, there is a theoretical risk of the whole syringe being delivered this way. However, this risk can be minimized (see 'Assembly' below).

2 The dose of analgesic delivered by the boost is wholly inadequate in relation to the recommended breakthrough pain rescue dose.

3 Drugs other than analgesics are usually present and bolus doses of these should not be given.

4 The delivery of a bolus dose can cause pain at the injection site.

5 The overall duration of the infusion is reduced, causing problems with renewal.

Indications

The use of CSCIs should **not** be considered the fourth step of the World Health Organization (WHO) pain ladder; intractable pain is not an indication. Additionally, use of the syringe driver should not be reserved solely for use in a dying patient—a CSCI can be considered when other routes of administration are inappropriate.

- ◆ Oral:
  - ▪ nausea and vomiting
  - ▪ dysphagia
  - ▪ severe weakness/unconsciousness
  - ▪ patient request (e.g. a large number of tablets)
- ◆ Rectal:
  - ▪ diarrhoea
  - ▪ bowel obstruction
  - ▪ patient preference (particularly the British)
- ◆ Intravenous/intramuscular:
  - ▪ cachexia
  - ▪ fear
  - ▪ discomfort

Assembly

The **length of liquid** within the syringe, not the volume, determines the rate of delivery with the syringe driver. The MS26 and MS16A can deliver a maximum length of 60 mm over 24 hours. This allows for greater flexibility in the choice of syringe (brand and size).

It is important to note that only Luer Lok™ syringes should be used. The maximum size of syringe that will fit on the driver is currently 35 ml. With this syringe size, a length of 60 mm equates to approximately 25 ml. Hence, the largest volume of liquid that can be infused is approximately 25 ml. This is important when considering large doses of certain drugs, for example, glycopyrronium (200 micrograms/ml) or midazolam (10 mg/2 ml).

Note

A 20 ml syringe is the **recommended minimum** for several reasons. Diluting the mixture to the maximum volume will reduce both the risks of adverse site reactions and incompatibility. In addition, the amount of drug lost in the infusion set will be reduced. Finally, the risk of abuse of the driver, through inappropriate use of the boost button, could be reduced; if too much fluid were to be forced through the driver, the occlusion alarm could potentially sound and the driver would stop infusing.

Procedure

1 Fill the syringe with drugs and dilute the mixture to a maximum length of 60 mm. Use the millimetre scale on the driver for reference.

2 Prime the infusion line, if required.

3 Measure the length of barrel against the millimetre scale on the syringe driver as shown in Fig. 3.

4 Set the delivery rate. This is derived by dividing the length of the barrel by the required infusion time. Examples are shown in the

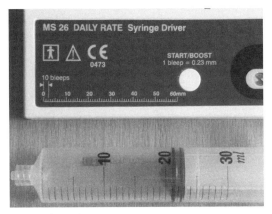

Fig. 3 Measuring the syringe.

table below. Note the infusion time for the **MS26** is calculated in **days**; the infusion time for the **MS16A** is calculated in **hours.**

Note: For practical reasons, when the MS16A is used for a 12 or 24 hour infusion, the desired barrel length is 48 mm.

Driver	Length of barrel	Duration of Infusion	Rate of Infusion
MS26	60 mm	24 hours (1 day)	60 mm/24 hours
	48 mm	12 hours (0.5 days)	96 mm/24 hours
MS16A	48 mm	24 hours	2 mm/hour
	48 mm	12 hours	4 mm/hour

Confusion between the two drivers, in relation to rate setting, has led to fatal errors. The MS26 is the easier of the two to use—for infusions over a 24-hour period, the length of the barrel represents the infusion rate. The MS26 offers a greater degree of flexibility in terms of volumes that can be infused since a longer length of solution, hence volume, can be administered (60 mm over 24 hours). For a 24-hour infusion, the maximum length for the MS16A would be 48 mm due to the practical maximum rate of 2 mm/h.

Risk management suggests the use of only one type of driver per site, preferably the MS26. There should be a programme of staff training and education within each unit using these devices. Additionally, and where possible, the syringe and contents should be regularly checked; an administration and checking record is suggested (see Appendix 1).

However, the sole use of one driver is not always possible. In situations where both drivers are employed, it would be prudent to fix the rate of infusion. For example, some centres that use both devices specify that the length of liquid is always 48 mm. The rates of infusion of both devices remain fixed at 48 mm/24 h (MS26) and 2 mm/h (MS16A).

5 The syringe is then attached to the driver as shown in Fig. 4.

6 The battery is then inserted. An audible alarm sounds. This is the noise the device makes when:

  ◆ The infusion has ended
  ◆ The line is blocked

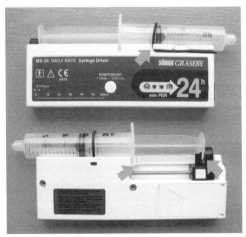

Fig. 4 Setting up the driver.

- The start/boost button is depressed for 10 seconds (MS26)
- The start/test button is held down for 5 seconds (MS16A)

7 Press the start button to silence the alarm and to activate the driv-er. If the light on the front of the driver does not flash (**MS26: every 25 seconds; MS16A: every second**), replace the battery. If, during the infusion, the light stops flashing, then the battery is almost depleted. However, the remaining contents in the syringe will be delivered, providing the duration of infusion does not exceed 24 hours. The battery can be replaced during the next assembly.

8 Finally, the clear plastic protective cover (as shown in Fig. 1) should be placed over the driver. At the time of writing, SIMS Graseby has developed a security device for these drivers (see Fig. 5). This 'lockbox' prevents accidental or intentional activation of the boost button and prevents tampering with the rate control. In the UK, however, such a device has not previously been thought necessary.

9 An alkaline 9 V battery, as recommended by SIMS Graseby, should be able to deliver 50 daily infusions.

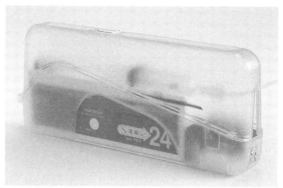

Fig. 5 SIMS Graseby MS Driver Lockbox

Siting the CSCI

The siting of the CSCI has implications for the patient. If the patient is ambulatory, then the chest or abdomen are the preferred sites. Previously, the upper aspect of the arm was considered first choice. However, movement of the arm may lead to the development of problems such as bruising. If the patient is distressed, the placement of the CSCI around the scapula will reduce the likelihood of the patient accidentally removing it. Occasionally, the thigh may be used.

Frequently asked questions

1 What diluent should be used to dilute drug mixtures?

In most cases, the diluent used should be *water for injections*. This is chosen for stability and solubility reasons. However, some mixtures need to be diluted with sodium chloride 0.9%; for example, mixtures containing methadone (see p. 24). Occasionally, dextrose 5% in water has been used. Chapters 2 and 4 describe, where applicable, the diluents that can be used.

2 When should the syringe driver be started?

When converting a patient from a modified release (m/r) preparation of an oral opioid (e.g. morphine, hydromorphone or oxycodone) to the syringe driver, there is no need for a crossover period; the driver may be started at the time of the next dose. For practical purposes, this is often the best method. However, in order to achieve or maintain adequate analgesia, it may be necessary to administer a suitable 'rescue' dose of subcutaneous opioid. Note that some centres will start the CSCI some 4 hours before the next oral dose was due.

If a CSCI is required for a patient on transdermal fentanyl, it is currently considered best practice to leave this *in situ*. Refer to Chapter 3 for further details.

3 When should the CSCI be stopped if oral treatment is to continue?

The CSCI should be stopped as soon as the oral m/r dose of opioid is given. No crossover period is necessary since the m/r preparations provide an 'immediate' release dose.

4 What is the usual number of drugs that can be mixed together?

Before mixing drugs together, it is important to check for stability information. This book has an extensive list of mixtures in Chapter 4; other sources of information include your local Medicines Information Centre (UK) or the Internet (e.g. www.palliativedrugs.com).

It is common to see at least two or three drugs mixed in the same syringe; occasionally four may be required. In fact, most of the symptoms encountered at the end of life can be controlled effectively by the use of only four drugs:

- Diamorphine (or morphine/hydromorphone)
- Midazolam
- Glycopyrronium (or hyoscine hydrobromide)
- Cyclizine

These drugs have been shown to be physically compatible at usual concentrations. (Refer to cyclizine and diamorphine monographs in Chapter 2 for known incompatibility issues.)

5 What can be done to minimize stability problems?

The mixture should be diluted to the maximum volume. The infusion should be delivered over a maximum time of 24 hours because chemical stability cannot be assured after this time. To further reduce the risk of incompatibility, the contents of the syringe driver and giving set should be protected from direct sunlight (especially mixtures containing levomepromazine). Temperature can also affect the stability of mixtures. Simple measures, such as ensuring the driver is placed on top of bed covers, rather than in them, can reduce the effects of temperature.

Certain incompatible mixtures are known to be dependent upon concentration (e.g. cyclizine and hyoscine butylbromide). The risk of crystallization or precipitation may be overcome by using more dilute 12-hourly infusions. However, to ensure that the rate setting is correct, consult a palliative care specialist in this situation.

6 What can be done do reduce site irritation?

Site irritation can occur with several drugs, such as cyclizine, levomepromazine, methadone and promethazine. In addition, patients may occasionally be allergic to the nickel needles. Site irritation can be reduced in several ways:

1 Dilute the mixture as much as practical; use a 12-hourly infusion rate if necessary; use saline 0.9% if applicable.

2 **Hyaluronidase** 1500 units can be injected into the site **prior** to the infusion if irritation is problematical. This needs to be done once per site only, not daily. Do not inject into an already inflamed site and do not mix in the syringe because degradation of hyaluronidase may occur over the 24 hours.

3 Although chemical evidence is lacking, clinical observations suggest 1 mg of **dexamethasone** added to the syringe may reduce site irritation, without affecting expected response. However, this may not always be practical since dexamethasone does render many mixtures incompatible (see Chapter 4).

4 Use of a Teflon or Vialon cannula may be useful in patients suffering excessive site irritation.

6 What can be done if a syringe driver is unavailable?

This is a fairly common problem encountered in hospitals in the UK. As a short-term measure, CSCIs can be administered by utilizing other syringe pumps, with the solution in the syringe being diluted to a suitable volume (e.g. 48 ml). These devices usually deliver at a rate of **millilitres per hour**. Alternatively, a butterfly needle may be sited subcutaneously and bolus injections can be given, as necessary, to cover the period until a driver becomes available. It would be wise to check with a palliative care specialist before proceeding.

Chapter 2

Drug Information

Introduction

During the last few years, it has become evident that a greater number of drugs are being administered by a continuous subcutaneous infusion (CSCI). The majority of these drugs (Table 1) are unlicensed for subcutaneous use, although most pharmaceutical companies will be aware that it occurs.

Most drug combinations used in palliative care form clear, colourless solutions that are free from precipitation or crystallization. This does not confirm stability because invisible chemical reactions may occur. For example, dexamethasone and glycopyrronium mix to form a clear, colourless solution that is free from precipitation. However, an unseen chemical reaction occurs and the effectiveness of the combination may be reduced considerably.

One of the most useful predictors of drug compatibility is pH. This can affect the solubility of drugs and chemical stability of the mixture. The majority of drugs given by CSCI are acidic, with only dexamethasone, diclofenac, ketorolac and phenobarbital being alkaline. Consequently, combinations involving these drugs tend to be incompatible and separate infusions are usually recommended. The pH values of individual drugs are included in the following sections. There are, however, several other factors that can affect the stability of drug mixtures, for example concentration, temperature and exposure to sunlight.

Table 1 Drugs that can be given by continuous subcutaneous infusion

Alfentanil	Dimenhydrinate	Hyoscine Hydrobromide	Morphine
Clonazepam	Fentanyl		Octreotide
Cyclizine	Glycopyrronium	Ketamine	Ondansetron
Dexamethasone	Haloperidol	Ketorolac	Phenobarbital
Diamorphine	Hydromorphone	Levomepromazine	Promethazine
Diclofenac	Hyoscine Butylbromide	Methadone	Ranitidine
Dihydrocodeine		Metoclopramide	Tramadol
		Midazolam	

Opioid analgesics

There are several opioid analgesics that can be administered via a CSCI. One of the commonly encountered problems involves the conversion of one opioid to another, for example, oral hydromorphone to subcutaneous diamorphine. Table 2 provides conversion factors from several different opioids and routes to subcutaneous diamorphine.[1–6, 38,42,64]

> **Important note** Equianalgesic doses are difficult to ascertain due to wide interpatient variations. Initial dose conversions should be conservative; it is preferable to under-dose the patient and use rescue medication for any shortfalls.

Table 2 Opioid conversion factors

Opioid (dose in milligrams)	Conversion factor to subcutaneous diamorphine* (in milligrams)
Alfentanil (parenteral)	10
Buprenorphine (oral)	16.7
Codeine (oral)	0.04
Diamorphine (oral)	0.33
Dihydrocodeine (oral)	0.04
Dihydrocodeine (subcutaneous)	0.15
Dipipanone (oral)	0.17
Fentanyl (parenteral)	30–50
Fentanyl (72 hour transdermal dose)	16.7 (for 24 hour dose equivalent)
Hydromorphone (oral)	2.5
Hydromorphone (parenteral)	5–6.6
Methadone (oral)	† (CSCI methadone preferred)
Morphine (oral)	0.33
Morphine (parenteral)	0.66–1.0
Oxycodone (oral)	0.66
Tramadol (oral and parenteral)	0.08

* Multiply the opioid dose (mg) by the conversion factor to give the equivalent subcutaneous diamorphine dose (mg).
  e.g. Fentanyl '25' patch
  = 25 µg/hour × 72
  = 1.8 mg fentanyl over 72 hours
  = 1.8mg × 16.7
  = 30mg diamorphine daily

† Methadone has a prolonged half-life that can result in accumulation with repeated doses. A palliative care or pain specialist should be consulted.

Diamorphine

Usual dose: There is no maximum dose of diamorphine in palliative care. A suitable starting dose via CSCI for an opioid-naïve patient would be 10 mg diamorphine. For patients with daily uncontrolled pain, the daily dose may be increased by 30–50%. Rescue doses for breakthrough pain should be prescribed and are calculated to be one-sixth of the total daily dose.

Preparations: 5 mg, 10 mg, 30 mg, 100 mg, 500 mg (UK).

Diluent: Dilute with water for injections. Saline 0.9% is not appropriate in most cases; avoid unless palliative care specialist states otherwise.

pH: 2.5–6.0. However, diamorphine is most stable within the pH range of 3.8–4.4 and with degradation increasing at neutral or basic pH values.[7] If diluted with saline 0.9%, the pH must remain below 6 in order for diamorphine to remain in solution.[8]

Information: Diamorphine is a derivative of morphine. *In vivo*, following subcutaneous injection, diamorphine is rapidly absorbed and converted to the active metabolite, 6-monoacetylmorphine. This metabolite is then slowly converted to morphine.

Following oral administration, diamorphine undergoes extensive first-pass metabolism to morphine. Both diamorphine and 6-monoacetylmorphine are more lipid soluble than morphine and consequently cross the blood–brain barrier more readily. Hence, diamorphine and morphine show similar oral potencies, but different parenteral values.[9]

The major excretory products of diamorphine metabolism are morphine-3-glucuronide (M3G, the principal metabolite) and morphine-6-glucuronide (M6G). Both M6G and M3G are renally excreted. Consequently, patients in renal failure are at a greater risk of developing diamorphine (or morphine) toxicity.[54] The adverse effects such as nausea, vomiting, drowsiness and respiratory depression have been attributed to accumulation of M6G. Similarly, adverse effects such as myoclonus, hyperalgesia and agitation have been attributed to the accumulation of M3G.[10] However, the exact pharmacological implications of these metabolites remain unknown.

Accumulation of diamorphine metabolites can pose problems, particularly as this is likely to occur as the patient's condition deteriorates and where any signs of diamorphine toxicity may be confused with general deterioration. The use of an opioid that is not renally excreted, or is metabolized to inactive compounds, would be more suitable, for example alfentanil. However, an empirical dose reduction of diamorphine of 30–50% may provide adequate analgesia, without the development of toxic effects.

Diamorphine is the opiate of choice in the UK for subcutaneous use due to its high solubility (1 g dissolves in 1.6 ml water compared with 1 g of morphine sulphate in 21 ml of water). The initial dose depends upon the patient's current opioid requirements. Approximate opioid equivalents are shown in Table 2. Note that there is great variation in the literature concerning equianalgesic doses.

Diamorphine hydrochloride and cyclizine lactate mixtures are chemically and physically stable in water for injections up to concentrations of 20 mg/ml over 24 hours. If the diamorphine concentration exceeds 20 mg/ml, crystallization may occur unless the concentration of cyclizine is no greater than 10 mg/ml. Similarly, if the concentration of cyclizine exceeds 20 mg/ml, crystallization may occur unless the concentration of diamorphine is no greater than 15 mg/ml.[11]

Diamorphine has also been shown to be physically and chemically stable with various concentrations of haloperidol, hyoscine butylbromide, hyoscine hydrobromide, metoclopramide, midazolam, octreotide and ondansetron.[12–16] Diamorphine and ketorolac mixtures in saline 0.9% have been shown to be physically compatible.[17] Finally, information within this book shows that diamorphine is physically compatible with clonazepam, dexamethasone, glycopyrronium and levomepromazine. See Chapter 4 for multiple drug compatibility data.

Morphine sulphate

Usual dose: There is no maximum dose of morphine in palliative care. A suitable starting dose via CSCI for an opioid-naïve patient would be 10–20 mg daily. If pain is uncontrolled, the dose can be increased by 30–50%. Rescue doses must be available for break-through pain and are calculated as one-sixth of the total daily dose.

Preparations: 10 mg/ml, 15 mg/ml, 20 mg/ml, 30 mg/ml (UK).

Diluent: Dilute with water for injections, or dextrose 5% in water. Saline 0.9% is not appropriate in most cases—avoid unless palliative care specialist states otherwise.

pH: 2.5–6.5. As with diamorphine, degradation increases at neutral or basic pH values.

Information: Orally, it is the opiate of choice for the treatment of moderate to severe cancer pain. Morphine is not widely administered in the UK via CSCI because of the availability of diamorphine. Nevertheless, where problems with the supply of diamorphine exist, morphine sulphate is an acceptable alternative. Morphine sulphate is used extensively in other areas of the world.

After subcutaneous injection, morphine is well absorbed and is predominantly metabolized in the liver to M3G (the principal metabolite) and M6G. The actual clinical implications of M6G and M3G have yet to be elucidated. However, it is believed that M6G is pharmacologically active and is more potent than morphine at the μ-receptor.[10] The major metabolite, M3G, is apparently devoid of analgesic activity and it has been suggested that it may actually antagonize the analgesic efficacy of morphine.[18]

Both M6G and M3G are renally excreted. Consequently, patients in renal failure are at a greater risk of developing morphine toxicity.[54] The adverse effects such as nausea, vomiting, drowsiness and respiratory depression have been attributed to the accumulation of M6G. Similarly, adverse effects such as myoclonus, hyperalgesia and agitation have been attributed to the accumulation of M3G.[10]

Accumulation of morphine metabolites can pose problems, particularly as this is likely to occur as the patient's condition deteriorates and where any signs of morphine toxicity may be confused with general deterioration. The use of an opioid that is not renally excreted, or is metabolized to inactive compounds, would be more suitable, for example alfentanil. However, an empirical dose reduction of morphine of 30–50% may provide adequate analgesia, without the development of toxic effects.

Subcutaneous morphine is considered to be 2–3 times as potent as oral morphine.[5,6,19] A range is stated because much of the analgesic activity of morphine is believed to be due to production of M6G,[20] a factor that varies between patients. Intravenous morphine is considered to be equipotent to subcutaneous morphine.[21] When converting from oral morphine to subcutaneous diamorphine, a ratio of 3 : 1 is commonly used.[1] The equianalgesic ratio for subcutaneous diamorphine to morphine is difficult to predict from the literature. Values suggested range from 1 : 1 to 2 : 3.

Morphine sulphate has been shown to be chemically and physically compatible with hyoscine hydrobromide, metoclopramide, midazolam and ondansetron.[22–24] Morphine sulphate has also been shown to be physically compatible with clonazepam, dexamethasone, dimenhydrinate, glycopyrronium, haloperidol (diluted with dextrose 5%), ketamine, ketorolac, levomepromazine, promethazine and ranitidine.[22,25,26] See Chapter 4 for multiple drug compatibility data.

Alfentanil

To be used only on the recommendation of a palliative care specialist

Usual dose: There is no maximum dose of alfentanil in palliative care. The initial dose depends upon the patient's previous opioid treatment (see Table 2 for diamorphine equivalents). For opioid-naïve patients, a suitable starting dose via CSCI would be 0.5–1 mg over 24 hours. If pain is uncontrolled, the dose can be increased by 30–50%. Rescue doses can be given for breakthrough pain. The optimum dosing schedule for breakthrough pain is presently unknown. Alfential has a very short duration of action and analgesia from a bolus dose may last for just 15-20 minutes. It is suggested that one sixth of the total daily dose is given every 2–3 hours. If more than three consecutive rescue doses are given for *breakthrough pain* at anytime the total daily dose should be increased by 30%. The net effect of this will be rapid titration of alfentanil which may necessitate two or more changes to the CSCI during a 24 hour period.

Preparations: 1 mg/2 ml; 5 mg/10 ml; 5 mg/ml.

Diluent: Dilute with water for injections or dextrose 5% in water. Saline 0.9% is not appropriate in most cases; avoid unless palliative care specialist states otherwise.

pH: 4.0–6.0.

Information: Alfentanil is a synthetic opioid, with strong agonist activity at μ- and k-opiate receptors. It is chemically related to fentanyl and is more lipophilic than morphine. Alfentanil is a suitable alternative to diamorphine for use in a CSCI, particularly in patients with renal failure. It is routinely used in surgical procedures as an analgesic and adjunct to general anaesthetics. Alfentanil is approximately **10 times** as potent as diamorphine (given subcutaneously)[3] and one-quarter as potent as fentanyl.[27]

Alfentanil is extensively metabolized in the liver to inactive compounds, with a mean elimination half-life of 90 minutes. The effects of coexisting liver disease may necessitate an empirical dosage reduction in order to avoid symptoms of opioid toxicity. A dosage reduction in obese patients may also be required. Dosage adjustments are usually **not** required in renal failure.[28,29]

One study[30] suggests that tolerance to the analgesic efficacy of alfentanil may develop relatively rapidly, which would limit its use in chronic treatment. However, a more recent study provided no evidence of tolerance to opioids.[31] Further work needs to be performed to determine the significance and incidence of this potential problem for all the opioids.

Alfentanil appears to be physically stable with most drugs used in the syringe driver (see Chapter 4) *except* cyclizine. As with diamorphine, the hydrochloride salt of alfentanil can cause crystallization with cyclizine as concentrations increase. Any mixtures with cyclizine should be diluted with water for injections and closely checked for signs of crystallization. Alfentanil has been shown to be physically and chemically compatible with midazolam[32] and ondansetron under stated conditions in saline 0.9%.[23]

Erythromycin and ketoconazole may increase alfentanil concentrations.

Dihydrocodeine

To be used only on the recommendation of a palliative care specialist. Note the injection is a controlled substance in the UK.

Usual dose: There is no maximum dose of dihydrocodeine in palliative care. Dihydrocodeine may be encountered via CSCI for use in patients with brain tumours. Breakthrough doses are calculated as a sixth of the total daily dose, although consideration should be given to the strength of preparation available.

Preparations: 50 mg/ml. Note that parenteral dihydrocodeine is a controlled drug in the UK.

Diluent: Dilute with water for injections. Saline 0.9% is not appropriate in most cases; avoid unless a palliative care specialist states otherwise.

pH: 3.0–4.5

Information: Dihydrocodeine is an analogue of codeine with weak opioid analgesic activity. There is no dose equivalence available between subcutaneous dihydrocodeine and diamorphine. Subcutaneous dihydrocodeine is approximately twice as potent as subcutaneous codeine[33] and 120 mg of intramuscular codeine is equivalent to 10 mg of intramuscular morphine.[34] Therefore, a conversion factor of **0.15** for subcutaneous dihydrocodeine to diamorphine appears reasonable (60 mg dihydrocodeine = 10 mg morphine = 6.6–10 mg diamorphine).

Dihydrocodeine is not usually given via CSCI, although its use has been reported in certain centres. It is reported to be stable with haloperidol and midazolam.[35]

Fentanyl

To be used only on the recommendation of a palliative care specialist.

Usual dose: There is no maximum dose of fentanyl in palliative care.

Preparations: 500 micrograms/10 ml; 100 micrograms/2 ml.

Diluent: Dilute with water for injections (for use with a syringe driver). Dextrose 5% in water may also be used.

pH: 4.0–7.5

Information: Fentanyl is unlikely to be administered via a CSCI using the syringe driver because the volumes involved are too great. There have, however, been several case reports documenting the efficacy of fentanyl infusions in cancer patients who were unable to tolerate morphine.[36–38]

Fentanyl is a synthetic opioid, chemically related to pethidine, with an action primarily at the μ-receptor. It is 50–100 times more potent than morphine and approximately four times as potent as alfentanil.[39] The main route of elimination is hepatic metabolism to inactive compounds, which are mainly excreted in the urine. Coexisting liver disease should not normally necessitate a change in dose;[9] however, an empirical dosage reduction may be required because fentanyl is extensively metabolized.

The metabolites of fentanyl are non-toxic and inactive. The use of fentanyl in patients with renal failure has not been associated with problems. Fentanyl could, therefore, be considered suitable for use in patients with low opioid requirements who are unable to tolerate diamorphine (or morphine), e.g. patients with renal failure where a dosage reduction of diamorphine does not produce the desired effect. It is, however, more expensive than diamorphine.

Equianalgesic ratios are difficult to determine. However, 10 mg of morphine is stated to be approximately equivalent to 150–200 micrograms of fentanyl in patients who had previously received opioids.[38,42] Therefore, when converting from subcutaneous diamorphine to fentanyl, an equianalgesic factor of **0.02–0.03** should be used.

Fentanyl citrate has been shown to be stable, under stated conditions, with dexamethasone, haloperidol, hyoscine butylbromide, ketorolac, levomepromazine, metoclopramide, midazolam and ondansetron.[15,26,40,41]

Hydromorphone

To be used only on the recommendation of a palliative care specialist.

Usual dose: There is no maximum dose of hydromorphone in palliative care. As with diamorphine, if pain is uncontrolled, the dose can be increased by 30–50%. Rescue doses should be available for breakthrough pain and are calculated as one-sixth of the total daily dose.

Preparations: 10 mg/ml, 20 mg/ml, 50 mg/ml.

Diluent: Dilute with water for injections (for use with a syringe driver). Dextrose 5% in water may also be used.

pH: 4.0–5.5.

Information: Hydromorphone is a semisynthetic derivative of morphine, with full opioid agonist properties. It is more soluble and potent than morphine and is particularly useful in countries where diamorphine is unavailable. This is ideal for CSCI, where small volumes are essential. Hydromorphone is therefore recommended for use in patients unable to tolerate morphine (outside the UK) or, in the absence of diamorphine, where large doses of morphine are involved. In the UK, hydromorphone injection is currently unavailable, except through 'special order' manufacturer, Martindale Pharmaceuticals Ltd in concentrations of 10 mg/ml, 20 mg/ml and 50 mg/ml. It should only be used via CSCI if diamorphine or alfentanil are considered inappropriate.

The adverse effect profile is similar to morphine. However, since the dose-limiting adverse effects of morphine may be due to the accumulation of the metabolites M6G and M3G,[10] problems such as nausea, vomiting and constipation may be less severe with hydromorphone.[43]

The main metabolite is hydromorphone-3-glucuronide, which is similar in structure to the morphine equivalent and is also renally excreted. If this metabolite accumulates, for example in patients with renal failure, symptoms such as neuroexcitation or hyperalgesia may occur.[44–46] However, a recent study suggests that hydromorphone is a safe and effective opioid in patients with renal failure.[47] Further work is necessary to determine the importance of this metabolite.

Experience of hydromorphone administration via CSCI is mainly limited to reports from Canada and the USA.[48–51] There is great variation in the literature concerning equianalgesia with hydromorphone. The oral to subcutaneous hydromorphone potency ratio ranges from 2.5 : 1 to 5 : 1. Subcutaneous hydromorphone is stated to be 15–20 times more potent than oral morphine.[5,6] It therefore follows that the equianalgesic ratio for subcutaneous hydromorphone to morphine is 1 : 7.5 to 1 : 10 and for diamorphine 1 : 5 to 1 : 6.6.

Hydromorphone has been shown to be physically and chemically stable with dimenhydrinate[52] and dexamethasone,[53] although this is concentration dependent in the latter case. Hydromorphone is chemically incompatible with hyaluronidase.[55]

Studies have shown hydromorphone to be physically stable with glycopyrronium, haloperidol, hyoscine hydrobromide, ketorolac, levomepromazine, metoclopramide, midazolam and phenobarbital.[26,56,57] See Chapter 4 for multiple drug compatibility data.

Methadone

To be initiated only in specialist palliative care centres.

Usual dose: There is no maximum dose of methadone. A CSCI must not be started in a methadone-naïve patient, unless under expert supervision. The dose depends upon the patient's previous oral methadone dose. Providing the patient has been successfully titrated with oral methadone, the total daily subcutaneous dose is estimated to be **50%** of the oral.[58] This can be given as a CSCI. Rescue doses for breakthrough pain are calculated as *one-sixth* of the total daily dose and are given *no more frequently than every 3 hours.* If two or more rescue doses are required, the total daily dose should be increased by 30%.

Preparations: 10 mg/ml, 20 mg/2 ml, 35 mg/3.5 ml, 50 mg/5 ml.

Diluent: Methadone should be diluted maximally in the syringe with saline 0.9%, although some centres use water or dextrose 5% in water.

pH: 4.5–7.0.

Information: Methadone is a synthetic opioid agonist with greater affinity than morphine for both δ- and μ-receptors. In addition, methadone exhibits non-competitive N-methyl-D-aspartate (NMDA) antagonist activity that may explain its suggested benefit in neuropathic pain.[58] It is readily absorbed following subcutaneous injection and is metabolized in the liver to inactive compounds that are excreted in bile and urine.

Hepatic impairment does not unduly affect methadone metabolism and dosage adjustments should not be necessary in stable disease states, although acute changes in hepatic function will require dosage adjustments. Dosage adjustments are not required for patients in renal failure, which allows methadone to be a suitable choice for use in patients who are unable to tolerate morphine.[9]

Methadone has a high bioavailability and very long elimination half-life of over 30 hours. This extremely long half-life shows wide interpatient variation and accumulation can occur with continuous use. Consequently, the dose of methadone is highly individualized.[59]

Methadone can cause severe irritation at the site of the infusion. Several methods for overcoming this problem have been suggested.[60,61] However, the following is recommended:

1 Usual diluent is saline 0.9%; dextrose 5% in water is occasionally used. In cases where local toxicity presents a problem and the mixture is believed to be hypertonic, water may be the best diluent.

2 Rotate the site every 2 days.

3 Some centres both in the UK and abroad recommend the use of 1 mg dexamethasone to be added to the syringe. This appears to attenuate local toxicity and the mixture appears to be physically stable (and the expected clinical outcome is observed). However, if other drugs are to be added to the syringe (such as glycopyrronium), dexamethasone can cause compatibility problems. In this case, inject the dexamethasone directly into the infusion site and flush with a small volume of water (e.g. 0.5 ml).

4 Hyaluronidase is an alternative to dexamethasone. It is used at a dose of 1500 units per site in patients experiencing local toxicity with methadone. Hyaluronidase must not be added to the syringe because it degrades over the 24-hour infusion period. It is injected directly into the site, prior to the infusion, via the butterfly needle and giving set. It should not be injected directly into an inflamed site.

Methadone has been shown to be physically compatible with dexamethasone, haloperidol, hyoscine butylbromide, ketorolac, levomepromazine, metoclopramide and midazolam.[26]

Carbamazepine, phenobarbital, phenytoin and **rifampicin** may reduce the effect of methadone; **cimetidine, fluoxetine** and **monoamine oxidase inhibitors** may increase the toxicity of methadone, so concomitant use should be avoided. Methadone may increase **zidovudine** levels.

Tramadol

To be used only on the recommendation of a palliative care specialist.

Usual dose: 200–600 mg over 24 hours; doses above 600 mg should be used cautiously. Breakthrough doses are calculated as one-sixth of the total daily dose.

Preparations: 100 mg/2 ml.

Diluent: Water for injections. Saline 0.9% and dextrose 5% in water may also be used.

pH: 6.0–6.8

Information: Tramadol is a synthetic compound that shows a weak affinity for the μ-receptor. The mode of action of tramadol is not completely understood, particularly since it has such weak opioid agonist activity. However, tramadol does inhibit the reuptake of noradrenaline and promotes the release of serotonin. Consequently, the analgesia produced by tramadol may involve the spinal modulation of pain through the activation of postsynaptic α_2-receptors.[62]

Tramadol is metabolized in the liver to form various metabolites; only one is pharmacologically active. The M1 metabolite has a greater affinity for the μ-receptor than tramadol. However, serum concentrations of M1 are no greater than 25%. Approximately 90% of tramadol and its metabolites are renally excreted. In moderate renal or hepatic impairment, the total daily dose should be halved.[63]

Tramadol is rarely administered via CSCI. Occasionally, however, patients may have obtained benefit from oral administration. It is in this group that tramadol via CSCI could be considered, especially if it has been used to treat bone pain. Equianalgesic ratios between subcutaneous tramadol and diamorphine do not exist. However, parenteral tramadol is stated to be approximately one-eighth as potent as parenteral morphine.[64] Hence a conversion ratio of 12.5 : 1 is suggested.

Clonazepam

Usual dose: 1–4 mg ov er 24 hours. Doses up to 8 mg can be used to treat terminal agitation. Clonazepam has a long half-life and may be given as a stat subcutaneous injection, rather than CSCI.

Diluent: Water for injections.

Preparations: 1 mg/ml in solvent with 1 ml water for injections to be added.

pH: 3.4–4.3.

Information: Clonazepam is a benzodiazepine derivative with antiepileptic properties. It is extensively metabolized in the liver to possibly weakly acting metabolites.[9] Clonazepam has several uses in palliative care:

- Neuropathic pain
- Terminal agitation
- Anxiety
- Myoclonus
- Seizures
- Intractable hiccup

Occasionally, a patient with neuropathic pain may require a syringe driver towards the end of life. Most recognized adjuvant analgesia cannot be given via CSCI. If left untreated, the neuropathic pain could manifest as terminal restlessness. Clonazepam can be used both orally and subcutaneously for the treatment of neuropathic pain. However, there are no randomized trials supporting the use of clonazepam in neuropathic pain or for administration via CSCI. Nonetheless, it is an accepted treatment in several centres and there are anecdotal reports in the literature.[65–68]

Clonazepam is an alternative to midazolam, but should be reserved for the treatment of terminal restlessness associated with a previous history of neuropathic pain, or where the volume of injection associated with midazolam is too great.

It has been shown that sorption into PVC infusion sets occurs with clonazepam injection.[69,70] The clinical significance of this effect is yet to be determined, although one study [69] suggests that this should be of little significance.

Reports suggest that clonazepam is physically compatible with haloperidol, hyoscine hydrobromide and morphine sulphate.[40,68] In addition, this book shows that clonazepam is physically stable with alfentanil, diamorphine, dexamethasone, glycopyrronium and methadone. See Chapter 4 for multiple drug compatibility data.

The use of drugs such as **phenobarbital** or **carbamazepine** may reduce the efficacy of clonazepam. The main adverse effect of clonazepam is drowsiness.

Cyclizine

Usual dose: 100–150 mg over 24 hours.

Diluent: Water for injections. Saline 0.9% must **not** be used.

Preparations: 50 mg/ml.

pH: 3.3–3.7.

Information: Cyclizine is an antihistamine with additional anti-muscarinic activity. It is metabolized in the liver to a relatively inactive metabolite.[9] It should be used with caution in patients with glaucoma, although this is not a contraindication for patients with advanced disease.

Cyclizine is a useful antiemetic if the cause of nausea or vomiting is due to stimulation of the vomiting centre (e.g. by radiotherapy to the head and neck, raised intracranial pressure) or vagus nerve (e.g. bowel obstruction with colic). It is also useful if nausea and vomiting is worse on movement.

This drug is implicated in many compatibility problems. Cyclizine may crystallise as the concentration of chloride ions increase or if the solution pH is greater than 6.8.[22] There is a theoretical risk of precipitation with drugs that are formulated in a solution containing chloride ions. Such drugs include alfentanil, diamorphine, ketamine, levomepromazine, metoclopramide, midazolam and ondansetron. In addition, there are known concentration-dependent compatibility issues with alfentanil, diamorphine, hyoscine butylbromide and metoclopramide.

Cyclizine lactate and diamorphine hydrochloride mixtures are chemically and physically stable in water for injections up to concentrations of 20 mg/ml over 24 hours. If the diamorphine concentration exceeds 20 mg/ml, crystallization may occur unless the concentration of cyclizine is no greater than 10 mg/ml. Similarly, if the concentration of cyclizine exceeds 20 mg/ml, crystallization may occur unless the concentration of diamorphine is no greater than 15 mg/ml.[11] Cyclizine forms a precipitate immediately when mixed with dexamethasone. See Chapter 4 for multiple drug compatibility data.

Adverse effects include drowsiness, dry mouth, urinary retention and restlessness. These are more common with higher doses. Rarely, aggravation of severe heart failure may occur and extrapyramidal reactions have also been reported. Cyclizine may occasionally cause irritation at the injection site.

Dexamethasone

Use with caution if a patient has a systemic infection or has had recent surgery.

Usual dose: 4–16 mg over 24 hours. Dexamethasone has a long half-life and therefore need only be given once daily, preferably in the morning. Most patients should be able to tolerate a single dose, but if central nervous system (CNS) disturbances occur, or if high doses are involved, dexamethasone should be given in divided doses or as a continuous infusion.

Diluent: Water for injections. May also be given in dextrose 5% in water, or in saline 0.9%.

Preparations: 8 mg/2 ml.

pH: Dexamethasone is formulated as the sodium phosphate salt. This has a pH from 7 to 8.5.

Information: Dexamethasone has several applications in palliative care, for example:

- Nausea and vomiting (due to intestinal obstruction or raised intracranial pressure).
- Raised intracranial pressure (caused by cerebral tumours, with symptoms of headache, nausea and vomiting, blurred vision and confusion).
- Breathlessness (secondary to tumour-induced airways obstruction).
- Pain (caused by nerve compression).
- Anorexia/cachexia (corticosteroids stimulate appetite).

Adverse effects include insomnia, delirium, restlessness and myopathy. Blood glucose levels can be raised, an effect not just limited to diabetic patients. Gastroprotective drugs should be considered if high doses are being used, or if a non-steroidal anti-inflammatory drug (NSAID) is co-prescribed (a proton pump inhibitor only).

Dexamethasone shows concentration-dependent physical and chemical compatibility with hydromorphone and ondansetron.[53,71]

Glycopyrronium chemically interacts with dexamethasone but no precipitate forms.[56] Therefore this combination must be avoided. Dexamethasone sodium phosphate is alkaline, so it is very likely to be incompatible with acidic solutions. Precipitation has occurred when mixed with cyclizine alone, haloperidol alone, and levomepromazine alone (see Chapter 4). Note that precipitation or lack of clinical efficacy has not been seen when diamorphine is included in mixtures containing dexamethasone and haloperidol or dexamethasone and cyclizine.

As much diluent as possible should be added to the mixture **before** the addition of dexamethasone. There may be transient turbidity with some mixtures, but a clear solution appears soon after. This only indicates a physical incompatibility if the turbidity remains.

Dexamethasone serum levels are reduced by **carbamazepine**, **phenobarbitone** and **phenytoin**. Higher doses may be necessary to successfully treat patients receiving these antiepileptics.

Diclofenac

To be used only on the recommendation of a palliative care specialist. Unless benefits outweigh risks, diclofenac must not be used if there is a history of recent peptic ulceration, gastrointestinal bleeding or hypersensitivity to aspirin or other NSAIDs.

Usual dose: 150 mg daily.

Diluent: Saline 0.9%. Must be given via a separate CSCI.

Preparations: 75 mg/3 ml.

pH: 7.8–9.0.

Information:

Diclofenac is currently one of two NSAID drugs that may be given via a CSCI. It must be used with caution in patients with renal impairment, although this is not an absolute contraindication in terminally ill patients.

NSAIDs are often used for the treatment of bone pain. Diclofenac is also a useful analgesic for biliary or renal colic. If the oral or rectal routes are unavailable, a CSCI may be considered. However, since a CSCI of diclofenac can cause irritation at the site of infusion, ketorolac should be considered. The irritation may be overcome by injecting the site with 1500 units of hyaluronidase or 1 mg of dexamethasone prior to the infusion.

When NSAIDs are given orally, the need for gastroprotection is deliberated, based upon recognized risk factors (e.g. age greater than 65 years, previous history of peptic ulcer or bleed or concurrent usage of aspirin, warfarin or corticosteroid).[72] However, if diclofenac is given via CSCI (it is assumed the oral route is inappropriate), the risk : benefit ratio of continued NSAID use must be discussed.

The adverse effect profile of diclofenac is similar to other NSAIDs; the clinically important adverse effects involve the gastrointestinal tract (ulceration, haemorrhage) and renal function (hyperkalaemia, uraemia, acute renal failure), which are more common in the elderly.

Dimenhydrinate

This drug is not available in the UK.

Usual dose: 50–200 mg over 24 hours. Stat doses of 25–50 mg can be given, but a dose of 400 mg should not normally be exceeded.

Diluent: Water for injections, dextrose 5% in water, or saline 0.9%.

Preparations: 50 mg/ml, 250 mg/5 ml, 500 mg/10 ml.

pH: 6.4–7.2.

Information: Dimenhydrinate consists of two moieties, diphenhydramine and 8-chlorotheophylline. It is believed that the pharmacological action of dimenhydrinate results from the diphenhydramine moiety. Like cyclizine, dimenhydrinate is both an antihistaminic and antimuscarinic. The pharmacokinetics of dimenhydrinate are poorly understood. Little is known about the absorption following a subcutaneous injection, or the elimination.

It should be used with caution in patients with *closed-angle* glaucoma or paralytic ileus due to the antimuscarinic effects. However, this is not a contraindication for patients with advanced disease.

Dimenhydrinate is a useful antiemetic if the cause of nausea or vomiting is due to stimulation of the vomiting centre (e.g. by radiotherapy to the head and neck, raised intracranial pressure) or vagus nerve (e.g. bowel obstruction with colic). Is also useful if nausea and vomiting is worse on movement.

Physical and chemical compatibility has been reported with hydromorphone[52] Dimenhydrinate is reportedly incompatible with glycopyrronium,[56] midazolam[102] phenobarbital and promethazine,[103] although anecdotally it has been successfully mixed with midazolam and a variety of other drugs, including morphine, haloperidol, metoclopramide, hyoscine butylbromide, hyoscine hydrobromide and octreotide.[104]

The adverse effects of dimenhydrinate are a result of its pharmacology. It is sedative, which can be beneficial, although, like hyoscine hydrobromide, it has the propensity to cause paradoxical agitation, usually at higher doses. Antimuscarinic effects, such as dry mouth can occur. There may also be pain at the injection/infusion site.

Glycopyrronium

Usual dose: From 600 micrograms to 2.4 mg over 24 hours. Stat doses of 200 micrograms may be given.

Diluent: Water for injections. Glycopyrronium may also be mixed with saline 0.9% and dextrose 5% in water.

Preparations: 200 micrograms/ml, 600 micrograms/3 ml.

pH: 2.3–4.3. The chemical stability of glycopyrronium is pH dependent. Above pH 6.0, the rate of hydrolysis increases significantly. Thus, glycopyrronium must not be added to mixtures where the pH is above this value. Addition of an alkaline drug (e.g. phenobarbital) can cause immediate precipitation.

Information: Glycopyrronium is an antimuscarinic agent with several potential uses in palliative care. As with all antimuscarinics, it should be avoided in patients with *closed-angle* glaucoma or paralytic ileus. However, this is not a contraindication for patients with advanced disease.

It is used in the treatment of excessive respiratory secretions and bowel colic. Glycopyrronium may be of benefit in the treatment of large-volume vomiting associated with bowel obstruction[73], possibly in combination with octreotide (authors' experience). It may also have a role as a treatment for excessive sweating. Glycopyrronium has been used to treat peptic ulcers.[74]

Glycopyrronium is preferred to hyoscine hydrobromide for the treatment of terminal secretions because:

1 It is less expensive and three times as potent[75].

2 It does not cross the blood–brain barrier so is devoid of CNS effects such as sedation and paradoxical agitation.

3 At normal doses, it has less of an effect on the ocular and cardiovascular systems than hyoscine hydrobromide.

Glycopyrronium does not relieve symptoms from already present secretions. It is imperative that treatment is initiated as soon as secretions become apparent.

Adverse effects are dose-related and are associated with its pharmacology. They include dry mouth, constipation and urinary retention. Unlike hyoscine hydrobromide, glycopyrronium can cause tachycardia. The effect of glycopyrronium may be enhanced in renal failure.[9]

Glycopyrronium chemically interacts with alkaline drugs. It reacts with dexamethasone but no precipitate forms. Immediate precipitation occurs with dimenhydrinate and phenobarbital.[56] Aside from these, glycopyrronium appears to be physically compatible with all other commonly used drugs. It has been shown to be chemically and physically compatible with ondansetron.[15] Glycopyrronium has also been shown to be physically compatible with hydromorphone, hyoscine hydrobromide, morphine and promethazine.[56] See Chapter 4 for multiple drug compatibility data.

Since glycopyrronium is only available in a 200 micrograms/ml concentration, the volume of injection may exceed the available syringe volume. In such cases, a 12-hourly infusion will have to be used.

Haloperidol

Usual dose: 2.5–10 mg over 24 hours (antiemetic); 10–30 mg over 24 hours (agitation). Haloperidol has a long half-life and may be given as a single bolus injection (up to doses of 10 mg).

Diluent: Water for injections. Dextrose 5% in water also used. Incompatible with saline 0.9%.

Preparations: 5 mg/ml.

pH: 3.0–3.6.

Information: Haloperidol is an antipsychotic agent, chemically related to chlorpromazine. It is a potent dopamine D_2-receptor antagonist. Haloperidol has minimal sedative properties at the low doses employed for nausea and vomiting. Higher doses are sedative and can be used to control agitation and confusion. However, at the doses required to produce sedation, there is an increased risk of extrapyramidal reactions. Clonazepam, levomepromazine or midazolam should be considered if sedation is required in such a patient. Haloperidol should not be used alone for terminal restlessness if myoclonus is present, since it lowers the seizure threshold.

It is useful when nausea and vomiting is due to stimulation of the chemoreceptor trigger zone, e.g. drugs (especially opioids), intestinal obstruction or hypercalcaemia. Haloperidol can also be used to treat hiccups.

Haloperidol has been shown to be chemically and physically compatible with diamorphine.[76] It has also been shown to be physically compatible with cyclizine, hydromorphone and morphine (in dextrose 5% in water).[25,57,77] See Chapter 4 for multiple drug compatibility data.

Extrapyramidal reactions may occur in the elderly, especially if other D_2-receptor antagonists are prescribed, e.g. **metoclopramide**, **levomepromazine**. **Fluoxetine** increases haloperidol serum levels and may lead to the development of extrapyramidal reactions; **carbamazepine** decreases serum levels.

Hyoscine butylbromide

Not to be confused with hyoscine *hydro*bromide.

Usual dose: 60–180 mg over 24 hours. Stat doses of 20 mg can be given.

Diluent: Water for injections.

Preparations: 20 mg/ml.

pH: 3.7–5.5.

Information: As for all antimuscarinic drugs, avoid in patients with *closed-angle* glaucoma or paralytic ileus. However, this is not a contraindication for patients with advanced disease.

Hyoscine butylbromide is mainly used for the treatment of intestinal colic associated with bowel obstruction. It can also be used to dry terminal secretions, although it is probably less effective than glycopyrronium or hyoscine hydrobromide. It does not readily cross the blood–brain barrier so is devoid of CNS effects such as sedation and paradoxical agitation.

Hyoscine butylbromide is also used in the treatment of large-volume vomiting that occurs with bowel obstruction.[93,96,98] It does not have a direct antiemetic effect, but does reduce gastrointestinal secretions. Bowel obstruction may lead to an increase in secretions, which can in turn precipitate nausea and vomiting. This effect of hyoscine butylbromide can be helpful in situations where large-volume vomiting is a problem.

Adverse effects include dry mouth, urinary retention and constipation.

Hyoscine butylbromide appears to be incompatible with cyclizine, although this reaction is concentration-dependent (see Chapter 4). The combination of hyoscine butylbromide and cyclizine is often favoured for the treatment of symptoms associated with bowel obstruction. In such cases, glycopyrronium should be used instead of hyoscine butylbromide. See Chapter 4 for multiple drug compatibility data.

Hyoscine hydrobromide

Not to be confused with hyoscine *butyl*bromide.

Usual dose: 800 micrograms to 2.4 mg over 24 hours. Stat doses of 400 micrograms can be given.

Diluent: Water for injections. Saline 0.9% and dextrose 5% in water may also be used.

Preparations: 400 micrograms/ml.

pH: 5.0–7.0.

Information: Hyoscine hydrobromide should be avoided in patients with *closed-angle* glaucoma or paralytic ileus. However, this is not a contraindication for patients with advanced disease.

Hyoscine previously had several uses in palliative care, which included:

- Antiemetic
- Colic associated with intestinal obstruction
- Bronchial secretions
- Sedation

Unfortunately, hyoscine hydrobromide can cause paradoxical agitation in addition to unwanted ocular and cardiovascular effects. Although the sedation provided by hyoscine hydrobromide can be beneficial, occasionally it is unwanted. For these reasons, glyco-pyrronium may be preferred for terminal secretions (and is more potent) and hyoscine butylbromide preferred for colic. Hyoscine hydrobromide is now rarely used for its sedative or antiemetic effects in palliative care in the UK.

Ketamine

To be used only on the recommendation of a palliative care specialist. Must not be used in patients with intracranial hypertension.

Usual dose: 60–360 mg over 24 hours.

Diluent: Saline 0.9% or dextrose 5% in water.

Preparations: 200 mg/20 ml, 500 mg/10 ml.

pH: 3.5–5.5.

Information: It must be used cautiously in patients with heart disease, especially hypertension, or those at risk of raised intraocular pressure.

Ketamine is a general anaesthetic, but at the subanaesthetic doses above, analgesia may be obtained with minimal sedation. Larger doses have been given,[78] but there is an increased risk of adverse effects.

It is believed to produce an analgesic effect through antagonism of the NMDA receptor.[79] Allodynia and hyperalgesia have been shown to be mediated via NMDA receptors. In patients who have developed these symptoms, or in patients with pain that is responding poorly to an adequate trial of opioids and common adjuvants, ketamine would be a suitable choice. *The dose of concurrent opioid must be reviewed because ketamine may restore responses to opioid analgesia, leading to opioid toxicity.*

Adverse effects include hallucinations, nightmares, confusion, delirium, tachycardia and increased blood pressure. Haloperidol (e.g. 5 mg over 24 hours) or benzodiazepines (e.g. midazolam) have been suggested to treat the vivid dreams or nightmares.[78] Note that there have only been case studies and no controlled trials reporting the effectiveness of ketamine in cancer pain.[79–82]

Ketamine has been shown to be chemically stable with midazolam when mixed in saline 0.9%.[83] In addition, ketamine has been shown to be physically stable when mixed with dexamethasone (low doses), diamorphine, haloperidol, ketorolac, levomepromazine, metoclopramide and morphine.[84,85]

Note that ketamine is only available in the UK for use in primary care on a named patient basis. The doctor completes a prescription as usual, but the pharmacist should contact the manufacturer to initiate supply.

Ketorolac

To be used only on the recommendation of a palliative care specialist. Must not be used if there has been recent peptic ulceration, gastrointestinal bleeding or hypersensitivity due to aspirin or other NSAIDs *unless* the benefits outweigh the risks.

Usual dose: 60–90mg over 24 hours.

Diluent: Saline 0.9% or dextrose 5% in water.

Preparations: 10 mg/ml, 30 mg/ml.

pH: pH 7.0–8.0.

Information: Ketorolac must be used with *extreme caution* in patients with moderate to severe renal failure, or in patients at risk of haemorrhage or incomplete haemostasis (e.g. liver disease).

Ketorolac is an NSAID with strong analgesic activity. It should only be used for bone pain where other NSAID formulations (e.g. diclofenac suppositories) are impractical or ineffective. Note that oral ketorolac has a direct irritant effect on the gastric mucosa in addition to the systemic effect. Therefore, subcutaneous ketorolac may be preferred. *Concurrent opioid dose should be reduced and other NSAIDs (if any) must be discontinued.*

There are no clinical trials to date involving the use of subcutaneous ketorolac in palliative care, only case studies.[17,85,86] A proton pump inhibitor (PPI) **must** be co-prescribed for prophylaxis against peptic ulceration. If oral treatment is impossible the addition of ranitidine to the CSCI may be considered, although it will provide less protection than a PPI. However, the risk : benefit ratio of using of ketorolac in the terminal stages of life without gastroprotective drugs would appear to be acceptable.

The adverse effect profile of ketorolac is similar to other NSAIDs; the clinically important adverse effects involve the gastrointestinal tract (ulceration, haemorrhage) and renal function (hyperkalaemia, uraemia, acute renal failure) that are more common in the elderly. Regular checks on renal function should be performed (if clinically indicated) because ketorolac-induced renal toxicity is associated with increasing levels of serum creatinine and potassium.[87]

Ketorolac has been shown to be physically stable in saline 0.9%, with diamorphine, dependent upon concentrations.[17] It is unlikely to be compatible with most drugs administered due to the alkaline pH. However, as shown in Chapter 4, it is physically compatible with ranitidine.

Levomepromazine (methotrimeprazine)

Usual dose: 6.25–25 mg over 24 hours (antiemetic); 25–200 mg over 24 hours (agitation). Irritation is possible at the infusion site. For lower doses (25–50 mg), a bolus subcutaneous injection can be given to overcome the problem. This is usually given at night. If an infusion is still required and irritation becomes a problem, hyaluronidase or low-dose dexamethasone (flush site before starting infusion due to incompatibility between dexamethasone and levomepromazine) can be injected into the site prior to starting the infusion.

Diluent: Water for injections. Saline 0.9% and dextrose 5% in water have also been used.

Preparations: 25 mg/ml.

pH: 4.5.

Information: Levomepromazine is a broad-spectrum antiemetic with a strong sedative effect. Note that a subcutaneous dose is believed to be twice as potent as that administered orally (i.e. 6.25 mg sc = 12.5 mg po). It acts on the main receptor sites involved in the vomiting pathway (dopamine D_2-receptors, serotonin 5-HT_2-receptors, histamine H_1-receptors and acetylcholine muscarinic receptors).

Doses above 50 mg/24 hours should be used cautiously in ambulatory patients because of the problems of sedation and postural hypotension. It is used at low doses to treat intractable nausea and vomiting. Levomepromazine has a long half-life and can be given as a single daily dose at night to avoid the problems of sedation.[88] At higher doses, it is a powerful sedative and can be used to treat terminal restlessness. However, if myoclonus is present, a benzodiazepine would be a more suitable choice, or should at least be included in the treatment regimen.

Levomepromazine is incompatible when mixed with dexamethasone. Solutions containing levomepromazine have developed a purple discoloration in ultraviolet light (i.e. sunlight) and should be discarded.[89] Levomepromazine has been shown to be physically compatible with methadone, morphine sulphate, hydromorphone and fentanyl[26] in addition to diamorphine and alfentanil (see Chapter 4).

Adverse effects include sedation, postural hypotension, dry mouth and extrapyramidal reactions (especially if other D_2-receptor antagonists are given). Hallucinations may occur rarely. Levomepromazine antagonizes the treatment of Parkinson's disease.

Metoclopramide

Must not be used if complete intestinal obstruction is present or suspected.

Usual dose: 30–120 mg over 24 hours.

Diluent: Water for injections. Saline 0.9% and dextrose 5% in water can also be used.

Preparations: 10 mg/2 ml.

pH: 3.0–5.0.

Information: Metoclopramide is a D_2-receptor antagonist, with non-sedating antiemetic and prokinetic properties. It is useful in the treatment of nausea and vomiting caused by drugs, gastric stasis or partial outflow obstruction. The inclusion of dexamethasone to the regimen in the latter two cases can improve the treatment of nausea and vomiting.

Extrapyramidal reactions can occur with metoclopramide, especially if other D_2-receptor antagonists (e.g. **haloperidol, levomepromazine**) are used. These reactions are more common in young females or the elderly. Doses of up to 60 mg are used regularly in palliative care and such reactions have rarely occurred. Metoclopramide antagonizes the treatment of Parkinson's disease.

Dosage reductions of up to 50% may be necessary in patients with moderate to severe renal impairment. An empirical dosage reduction may be necessary in patients with a significant degree of hepatic impairment.[9] Antimuscarinic drugs can directly interfere with the prokinetic action and concurrent use should be avoided. For example, when used with **cyclizine** or **dimenhydrinate**, higher doses of metoclopramide may be required to achieve the desired effect.

Metoclopramide can cause irritation at the site of injection. Due to the presence of chloride ions in the injection, crystallization *may* occur with cyclizine. The injection should be discarded if it discolours. Metoclopramide has been shown to be physically and chemically compatible with diamorphine and morphine.[12,22] In addition, it has been shown to be physically compatible with dexamethasone sodium phosphate,[22] alfentanil (see Chapter 4), fentanyl, hydromorphone and methadone.[26]

Midazolam

Usual dose: 10–60 mg over 24 hours for seizures, anxiety or terminal agitation. If agitation is poorly controlled at this maximum dose, the additional use of levomepromazine should be considered. Clonazepam or phenobarbital may be considered for control of seizures.

Diluent: Water for injections. Saline 0.9% and dextrose 5% in water may also be used.

Preparations: 10 mg/2 ml.

pH: 2.9–3.7.

Information: Midazolam is a short-acting benzodiazepine, which is suitable for CSCI. It is metabolized in the liver mainly to a less active metabolite. All metabolites are excreted in the urine. Empirical dosage reductions may be necessary in liver disease (main site of metabolism) and renal disease (accumulation of metabolite).[9]

As for clonazepam, midazolam has several uses in palliative care:

- Terminal agitation
- Myoclonus
- Seizures
- Intractable hiccup
- Anxiety

Unlike clonazepam, midazolam has not been shown to be of benefit in neuropathic pain. Midazolam is preferred to clonazepam in emergency situations, such as major haemorrhage, because of its quicker onset of action. Although indicated for the treatment of hiccups, midazolam has been implicated as a cause of drug-induced hiccups.[90]

Midazolam has been shown to be physically and chemically compatible with alfentanil,[32] diamorphine,[13] morphine sulphate[22] and ondansetron.[23] It is incompatible with dimenhydrinate.[102]

Tolerance has been reported to develop rapidly (within a week) to the effects of midazolam, requiring increasing doses, or the introduction of another drug.[91]

Octreotide

To be used only on the recommendation of a palliative care specialist.

Usual dose: 300–600 micrograms over 24 hours.

Diluent: Saline 0.9% is the recommended diluent. Water or dextrose 5% in water can also be used.

Preparations: 50 micrograms/ml, 100 micrograms/ml, 500 micrograms/ml.

pH: 3.9–4.5.

Information: Octreotide is a somatostatin analogue that has potentially several roles in palliative care. One of its actions involves the reduction of intestinal secretions of water and sodium, in addition to stimulating the absorption of water and electrolytes. It is, therefore, useful in situations where excessive diarrhoea (e.g. carcinoid syndrome) or large-volume vomiting are problematical.

Octreotide has an as yet undefined role in the management of gastrointestinal obstruction. It is an expensive drug and should not be used routinely to treat this condition. There have been several case reports of the effectiveness of octreotide,[92–95] and one small controlled trial.[96] Doses above 600 micrograms are not thought to provide further benefit,[97] although some centres will continue to use over 1000 micrograms. Combination with an antimuscarinic drug such as hyoscine butylbromide[98] or glycopyrronium (authors' experience) may further improve symptom control.

In the absence of stability data it would be wise to administer octreotide either as a separate CSCI, or as a bolus subcutaneous injection. In the latter case, the ampoule should be warmed prior to injection to reduce pain on administration.

Octreotide has been shown to be physically and chemically compatible with diamorphine.[14] Chapter 4 provides additional information regarding the physical stability of multiple drug combinations.

Adverse effects include dry mouth (although tolerance should develop) and flatulence (reduce dose and increase slowly).

Ondansetron

To be used only on the recommendation of a palliative care specialist.

Usual dose: 24 mg over 24 hours. Up to 32 mg may be given.

Diluent: Water for injections. Saline 0.9% and dextrose 5% in water can also be used.

Preparations: 4 mg/2 ml, 8 mg/4 ml.

pH: 3.3–4.0. Ondansetron may precipitate with alkaline drugs.

Information: It is a selective 5-HT$_3$ antagonist with proven efficacy in the treatment of acute nausea and vomiting associated with radiotherapy to the upper abdomen, and chemotherapy. Nonetheless, the place of 5-HT$_3$ antagonists in palliative medicine remains to be determined. There have been several case reports[99,100] stating good results in patients unresponsive to conventional antiemetic treatment. In addition, ondansetron has been shown to be beneficial in patients with pruritus due to cholestasis.[101] The main adverse effect is constipation. Consequently, ondansetron may be of benefit in treating the diarrhoea associated with carcinoid syndrome.

Serotonin (5-HT) is released by enterochromaffin cells in the bowel wall in response to certain stimuli, in particular bowel distension. 5-HT is also released as a result of kidney damage. Ondansetron may be a suitable third- or fourth-line treatment in patients with distension or renal damage who have failed to respond to conventional antiemetics. The dose should be reduced in severe liver disease.

There is limited stability data available, but ondansetron is compatible with diamorphine (in saline 0.9%) at concentrations up to 0.64 mg/ml and 5 mg/ml, respectively.[16] Studies have shown ondansetron to be physically and chemically compatible with alfentanil, dexamethasone (high concentrations are likely to be incompatible), fentanyl, glycopyrronium, midazolam, metoclopramide and morphine sulphate.[15,71]

Phenobarbital (phenobarbitone)

To be used only on the recommendation of a palliative care specialist. Note this is a controlled substance in the UK.

Usual dose: 200–600 mg over 24 hours. Higher doses up to 1200 mg have been used. Bolus doses between 50 mg and 200 mg can be given, but may be painful (see pH below).

Diluent: Water for injections, or saline 0.9%.

Preparations: 30 mg/ml, 60 mg/ml, 200 mg/ml.

pH: 10.0–11.0. Subcutaneous bolus injections can cause tissue necrosis due to the high pH. However, a CSCI is usually well tolerated.

Information: Phenobarbital is a long-acting barbiturate. It may be useful in palliative care as an antiepileptic. If a patient is unable to take oral anticonvulsants, and a benzodiazepine is ineffective or impractical, phenobarbital can be given for epilepsy prophylaxis/treatment. In addition, phenobarbital can be given to treat refractory terminal restlessness.

It is formulated at an alkaline pH and is therefore unlikely to be stable with most drugs. It should be given via separate driver.

Promethazine

To be used only on the recommendation of a palliative care specialist.

Usual dose: 50–150 mg over 24 hours. Stat doses of 25–50 mg can be given.

Diluent: Water for injections, dextrose 5% in water and saline 0.9%.

Preparations: 25 mg/ml.

pH: 4.0–5.5. Probably incompatible with alkaline drugs.

Information: Promethazine is a useful drug, having antihistaminic, antimuscarinic and antidopaminergic properties. These pharmacological actions confer useful antiemetic and sedative properties. It is metabolized in the liver. Promethazine should be used with caution in patients with glaucoma or paralytic ileus, although this is not a contraindication for patients with advanced disease.

Promethazine can be considered as an antiemetic if the cause of nausea or vomiting is due to stimulation of the vomiting centre (e.g. by radiotherapy to the head and neck, raised intracranial pressure), vagus nerve (e.g. bowel obstruction with colic), chemoreceptor trigger zone (e.g. drugs, hypercalcaemia, bowel obstruction) or is worse on movement.

Promethazine is incompatible with dimenhydrinate (although there should be no need to co-prescribe these drugs).[103] It is also incompatible with ketorolac.[105] Promethazine has been shown to be physically compatible with glycopyrronium.[56] Anecdotally, it has been reported to mix with morphine sulphate and precipitate with midazolam.[106]

The adverse effects of promethazine are a result of its pharmacology. It is a sedative, which can be beneficial, although like hyoscine hydrobromide, it has the propensity to cause paradoxical agitation, usually at higher doses. Antimuscarinic effects, such as dry mouth, can occur. Extrapyramidal reactions can also occur; again these may occur at higher doses. Sterile abscesses or necrotic lesions have been reported on rare occasions following subcutaneous use of promethazine. However, anecdotal evidence suggests that a CSCI of promethazine is both effective and well tolerated.[106]

Ranitidine

To be used only on the recommendation of a palliative care specialist.

Usual dose: 150–300 mg over 24 hours.

Preparations: 50 mg/2 ml.

Diluent: Water for injections. Dextrose 5% in water and saline 0.9% can also be used.

pH: 6.7 to 7.3.

Information: The H_2-antagonists reduce both gastric acid output and the volume of gastric secretions. Although not as effective as the proton pump inhibitors, ranitidine may afford some protection against NSAID-induced peptic ulceration and reduce the symptoms of dyspepsia that may occur. Ranitidine can be infused concurrently with ketorolac (see Chapter 4). Note, however, there is no evidence to suggest that a CSCI of ranitidine will prevent NSAID-induced gastroduodenal damage.

Ranitidine is incompatible with midazolam and phenobarbital.[22]

References

1. Regnard CFB, Tempest S. *A Guide to Symptom Relief in Advanced Cancer*, 4th edn. Hochland & Hochland Ltd, Hale;1998.
2. Cherry NI. Opioid analgesics. Comparative features and prescribing guidelines. *Drugs* 1996; **51** (5): 713–737.
3. Kirkham SR, Pugh R. Opioid analgesia in uraemic patients. *Lancet* 1995; **345**: 1185.
4. Doyle D, Hanks GWC, MacDonald N (eds). *Oxford Textbook of Palliative Medicine*, 2nd edn. Oxford University Press, Oxford; 1998.
5. Levy MH. Pharmacologic treatment of cancer pain. *N Engl J Med* 1996; **335** (15): 1124–1132.
6. Lothian ST, Fotis MA, Von Gunten CF *et al.* Cancer pain management through a pharmacist-based analgesic dosing service. *Am J Health Syst Pharm* 1999; **56**: 1119–1125.
7. Beaumont IM. Stability study of aqueous solutions of diamorphine and morphine using HPLC. *Pharm J* 1982; **229**: 39–41
8. Kirk B, Hain WR. Diamorphine injection BP incompatibility. *Pharm J* 1985; **235**: 171.
9. Parfitt K (ed.). *Martindale: The Extra Pharmacopoeia*, 32nd edn. Pharmaceutical Pres, London; 1999.
10. Mercadante S. The role of morphine glucuronides in cancer pain. *Palliat Med* 1999; **13**: 95–104.
11. Grassby PF, Hutchings L. Drug combinations in syringe drivers: the compatibility and stability of diamorphine with cyclizine and haloperidol. *Palliat Med* 1997; **11**: 217–224.
12. Regnard C, Pashley S, Westrope F. Anti-emetic/diamorphine mixture compatibility in infusion pumps. *Br J Pharm Pract* 1986; **8**: 218–220.
13. Allwood MC, Brown PW, Lee M. Stability of injections containing diamorphine and midazolam in plastic syringes. *Int J Pharm Pract* 1994; **3**: 57–59.
14. Fielding H, Kyaterekera N, Skellern GG *et al.* The compatibility of octreotide acetate in the presence of diamorphine hydrochloride in polypropylene syringes. *Palliat Med* 2000; **14** (3) :205–207.
15. Stewart JT, Warren FW, King DT *et al.* Stability of ondansetron hydrochloride and 12 medications in plastic syringes. *Am J Health Syst Pharm* 1998; **55**: 2630–2634.
16. Data on file. GlaxoSmithKline UK Ltd.
17. Hughes A, Wilcock A, Corcoran R. Ketorolac: continuous subcutaneous infusion for cancer pain. *J Pain Symp Manage* 1997; **13** (6): 315.
18. Smith GD, Smith MT. Morphine-3-glucuronide: evidence to support its putative role in the development of tolerance to the antinociceptive effects of morphine in rat. *Pain* 1995: **52**: 51–60.

19. Hanks GW, De Conno F, Ripamonti C *et al.* Morphine in cancer pain: modes of administration. *Br Med J* 1996; **312**: 823–826.

20. Hanks GW, Hoskin PJ, Aherne GW *et al.* Explanation for potency of repeated oral doses of morphine? *Lancet* 1987; **2**: 723–725.

21. Nelson KA, Glare PJ, Walsh D, Groh ES. A prospective, within patient, crossover study of continuous intravenous and subcutaneous morphine for chronic cancer pain. *J Pain Symp Manage* 1997; **13**: 262–267.

22. Trissel LA. *Handbook on Injectable Drugs*, 11th edn. American Society of Health System Pharmacists Bethesda; 2000

23. Stewart JT, Warren FW, King DT *et al.* Stability of ondansetron hydrochloride and 12 medications in plastic syringes. *Am J Health Syst Pharm* 1998; **55**: 2630–2634.

24. Trissel LA, Xu Q, Martinez JF, Fox JL. Compatibility and stability of ondansetron hydrochloride with morphine sulphate and with hydromorphone hydrochloride in 0.9% sodium chloride injection at 4, 22 and 32 degrees C. *Am J Hosp Pharm* 1994; **51** (17): 2138–2142.

25. Lau MH, Hackman C, Morgan DJ. Compatibility of ketamine and morphine injections. *Pain* 1998; **75**: 389–390.

26. Chandler SW, Trissel LA, Weinstein SM. Combined administration of opioids with selected drugs to manage pain and other cancer symptoms: initial safety screening for compatibility. *J Pain Symp Manage* 1996; **12**: 168–171.

27. Larijani GE, Goldberg ME. Alfentanil hydrochloride: a new short acting narcotic analgesic for surgical procedures. *Clin Pharm* 1987; **6**: 275–282.

28. Tegeder I, Lotsch J, Geisslinger G. Pharmacokinetics of opioids in liver disease. *Clin Pharmacokinet* 1999; **37**: 17–40.

29. Maitre PO, Vozeh S, Heykants J *et al.* Population pharmacokinetics of alfentanil: the average dose–plasma concentration relationship and interindividual variability in patients. *Anaesthesiology* 1987; **66**: 3–12.

30. Hill HF, Coda BA, Mackie AM, Iverson K. Patient controlled analgesic infusions: alfentanil versus morphine. *Pain* 1992; **49**: 301–310.

31. Schragg S, Checketts MR, Kenny GN. Lack of rapid development of opioid toxicity during alfentanil and remifentanil infusions for post-operative pain. *Anesth Analg* 1999; **89**: 753–757.

32. Mehta AC, Kay EA. Storage time can now be extended. *Pharm Pract* 1997; **7**: 305–308.

33. Dollery CT (ed.). *Therapeutic Drugs*. Churchill Livingstone, Edinburgh; 1991.

34. Woodruff R. *Cancer Pain*. Asperula Pty Ltd, Victoria, Australia; 1997.

35. Bradley K. Swap data on drug compatibilities. *Pharmacy Pract* 1996; **6**: 69–72.

36. Mercadante S, Caligara M, Sapio M *et al.* Subcutaneous fentanyl infusion in a patient with bowel obstruction and renal failure. *J Pain Symp Manage* 1997; **13**: 241–244.

37. Lenz KL, Dunlap DS. Continuous fentanyl infusion: use in severe cancer pain. *Ann Pharmacother* 1998; **32**: 316–319.

38. Paix A, Coleman A, Lees J *et al.* Subcutaneous fentanyl and sufentanil infusion substitution for morphine intolerance in cancer pain management. *Pain* 1995; **63**: 263–269.

39. Clotz MA, Nahata MC. Clinical uses of fentanyl, sufentanil and alfentanil. *Clin Pharm* 1991; **10**: 581–593.

40. Drummond SH, Peterson GM, Galloway JG, Keefe PA. National survey of drug use in palliative care. *Palliat Med* 1996; **10**: 119–124.

41. Wilson KM, Schneider JJ, Ravenscroft PJ. Stability of midazolam and fentanyl infusion solutions. *J Pain Symp Manage* 1998; **16**: 52–58.

42. Hunt R, Fazekas B, Thorne D, Brooksbank M. A comparison of subcutaneous morphine and fentanyl in hospice cancer patients. *J Pain Symp Manage* 1999; **18**: 111–119.

43. De Stoutz ND, Bruera E, Suarez-Almozor M. Opioid rotation for toxicity reduction in terminal cancer patients. *J Pain Symp Manage* 1995; **10**: 378–384.

44. Babul N, Darke AC. Putative role of hydromorphone metabolites in myoclonus. *Pain* 1992; **51**: 260–261.

45. Babul N, Darke AC, Hagen N. Hydromorphone metabolite accumulation in renal failure. *J Pain Symp Manage* 1995; **10**: 184–186.

46. Smith MT. Neuroexcitatory effects of morphine and hydromorphone: evidence implicating the 3-glucuronide metabolites. *Clin Exp Pharmacol Physiol* 2000; **27**: 524–528.

47. Lee MA, Leng MEF, Tiernan EJJ. Retrospective study of the use of hydromorphone in palliative care patients with normal and abnormal urea and creatinine. *Palliat Med* 2001; **15**: 26–34.

48. Lawler P, Turner K, Hanson J, Bruera E. Dose ratio between morphine and hydromorphone in patients with cancer: a retrospective study. *Pain* 1997; **72**: 79–85.

49. Bruera E, Pereira J, Watanabe S *et al.* Opioid rotation in patients with cancer pain. A retrospective comparison of dose ratios between methadone, hydromorphone and morphine. *Cancer* 1996; **78** (4): 852–857.

50. Storey P, Hill HH, St Louis RH *et al.* Subcutaneous infusions for the control of cancer symptoms. *J Pain Symp Manage* 1990; **5** (1): 33–41.

51. Miller MG, McCarthy N, O'Boyle CA, Kearney M. Continuous subcutaneous infusion of morphine vs. hydromorphone: a controlled trial. *J Pain Symp Manage* 1999; **18** (1): 9–16.

52. Walker SE, Iazzetta J, De Angelis C, Lau DCW. Stability and compatibility of combinations of hydromorphone and dimenhydrinate, lorazepam or prochlorperazine. *Can J Hosp Pharm* 1993; **46**: 61–65.

53. Walker SE, De Angelis C, Iazzetta J, Eppel JG. Compatibility of dexamethasone sodium phosphate with hydromorphone hydrochloride or diphenhydramine hydrochloride. *Am J Hosp Pharm* 1991; **48** (10): 2161–2166.

54. Peterson GM, Randall CT, Paterson J. Plasma levels of morphine and morphine glucuronides in the treatment of cancer pain: relationship to renal function and route of administration. *Eur J Clin Pharmacol* 1990; **38** (2): 121–124.

55. Walker SE, Lau DWC. Compatibility and stability of hyaluronidase and hydromorphone. *Can J Hosp Pharm* 1992; **45**: 187–192.

56. Ingallinera TS, Kapadia AJ, Hagman D, Klioze O. Compatibility of glycopyrrolate injection with commonly used infusion solutions and additives. *Am J Hosp Pharm* 1979; **36** (4): 508–510.

57. Huang E, Anderson RP. Compatibility of hydromorphone hydrochloride with haloperidol lactate and ketorolac tromethamine. *Am J Hosp Pharm* 1994; **51** (23): 2963.

58. Gannon C. The use of methadone in the care of the dying. *Eur J Palliat Care* 1997; **4**: 152–158.

59. Fitzgibbon DR, Ready LB. Intravenous high-dose methadone administered by patient controlled analgesia and continuous infusion for the treatment of cancer pain refractory to high-dose morphine. *Pain* 1997; **73**: 259–261.

60. Mathew P, Storey P. Subcutaneous methadone in terminally ill patients: manageable local toxicity. *J Pain Symp Manage* 1999; **18** (1): 49–52.

61. Makin M, Morley JS. Subcutaneous methadone in terminally ill patients (letter). *J Pain Symp Manage* 2000; **19** (4): 237–238.

62. Duthie DJR. Remifentanil and tramadol. *Br J Anaesth* 1998; **81**: 51–57.

63. Bamigbade TA, Langford RM. The clinical use of tramadol hydrochloride. *Pain Rev* 1998; **5**: 155–182.

64. Silvasti M, Svartling N, Pitkanen M, Rosenberg PH. Comparison of intravenous patient controlled analgesia with tramadol versus morphine after microvascular breast reconstruction. *Eur J Anaesthesiol* 2000; **17** (7): 448–455.

65. Glynn C. An approach to the management of the patient with deafferentation pain. *Palliat Med* 1989; **3**: 13–21.

66. Bartusch SL, Sanders BJ, D'Alessio JG, Jernigan JR. Clonazepam for the treatment of lancinating phantom limb pain. *Clin J Pain* 1996; **12**: 59–62.

67. Reddy S, Patt RB. The benzodiazepines as adjuvant analgesics. *J Pain Symp Manage* 1994; **9**: 510–514.

68. Burke AL. Palliative care: an update on terminal restlessness. *Med J Aust* 1997; **166**: 39–42.

69. Nation RL, Hackett LP, Dusci LJ. Uptake of clonazepam by plastic intravenous infusion bags and administration sets. *Am J Hosp Pharm* 1983; **40**: 1692–1693.

70. Hooymans PM, Janknegt R, Lohman JJ. Comparison of clonazepam sorption to polyvinyl chloride-coated and polyethylene-coated tubings. *Pharm Weekbl* 1990; **12**: 188–189.

71. Hagan RL, Mallett MS, Fox JL. Stability of ondansetron hydrochloride and dexamethasone sodium phosphate in infusion bags and syringes for 32 days. *Am J Health Syst Pharm* 1996; **53**: 1431–1435.

72. Koch M, Dezi A, Tarquini M, Capurso L Prevention of non-steroidal anti-inflammatory drug-induced gastrointestinal mucosal injury: risk factors for serious complications. *Dig Liver Dis* 2000; **32** (2): 138–151.

73. Davis MP, Furste A. Glycopyrrolate: a useful drug in the palliation of mechanical bowel obstruction. *J Pain Symp Manage* 1999; **18**: 153–154.

74. Dollery CT (ed.). *Therapeutic Drugs*. Churchill Livingstone, Edinburgh; 1991.

75. Twycross R. *Symptom Management in Advanced Cancer*, 2nd edn. Radcliffe Medical Press, Oxford; 1997.

76. Allwood MC. The stability of diamorphine alone and in combination with anti-emetics in plastic syringes. *Palliat Med* 1991; **5**: 330–333.

77. Fawcett JP, Woods DJ, Munasiri B, Becket G. Compatibility of cyclizine lactate and haloperidol lactate. *Am J Hosp Pharm* 1994; **51**: 2292.

78. Fallon MT, Welsh J. The role of ketamine in pain control. *Eur J Palliat Care* 1996; **3** (4): 143–146.

79. Mercadante S, Lodi F, Sapio M *et al.* Long term ketamine subcutaneous infusion in neuropathic cancer pain. *J Pain Symp Manage* 1995; **10**: 564–568.

80. Wood T, Sloan R. Successful use of ketamine for central pain. *Palliat Med.* 1997; **11**: 57–58.

81. Fine PG. Low dose ketamine for the management of opioid non-responsive terminal cancer pain. *J Pain Symp Manage* 1999; **17**: 296–300.

82. Lloyd-Williams M. Ketamine for cancer pain. *J Pain Symp Manage* 2000; **19**: 79–80.

83. Lechner MD, Kreuscher H. Chemical compatibility of ketamine and midazolam in infusion solutions. *Anaesthetist* 1990; **39** (1): 62–65.

84. Lau MH, Hackman C, Morgan DJ. Compatibility of ketamine and morphine injections. *Pain* 1998; **75**: 389–390.

85. Blackwell N, Bangham L, Hughes M *et al.* Subcutaneous ketorolac—a new development in pain control. *Palliat Med* 1993; **7**: 63–65.

86. De Conno F, Zecca E, Martini C *et al.* Tolerability of ketorolac administered via continuous subcutaneous infusion for cancer pain: a preliminary report. *J Pain Symp Manage* 1994; **9**: 119–121.

87. Gillis JC, Brogden RN. Ketorolac. A reappraisal of its pharmacodynamic and pharmacokinetic properties and therapeutic use in pain management. *Drugs* 1997; **53** (1): 139–188.

88. Twycross RG, Barkby GD, Hallwood PM. The use of low dose methotrimeprazine (levomepromazine) in the management of nausea and vomiting. *Prog Palliat Care* 1997; **5** (2): 49–53.

89. Davies A, Mitchell M. Methotrimeprazine and UV light. *Palliat Med* 1996; **10**: 264.

90. Thompson DF, Landry JP. Drug-induced hiccups. *Ann Pharmacother* 1997; **31**: 367–369.

91. Bottomley DM, Hanks GW. Subcutaneous midazolam in palliative care. *J Pain Symp Manage* 1990; **5**: 259–261.

92. Mercadante S, Spoldi E, Caraceni A *et al.* Octreotide in relieving gastrointestinal symptoms due to bowel obstruction. *Palliat Med* 1993; **7**: 295–299.

93. Ripamonti C. Management of bowel obstruction in advanced cancer patients. *J Pain Symp Manage* 1994; **9**: 193–200.

94. Mangili G, Franchi M, Mariani M *et al.* Octreotide in the management of bowel obstruction in terminal ovarian cancer. *Gynecol Oncol* 1996; **61** (3): 345–348.

95. Mercadante S, Kargor J, Nicolosi G. Octreotide may prevent definite intestinal obstruction. *J Pain Symp Manage* 1997; **13** (6): 352–355.

96. Ripamonti C, Mercadante S, Groff L *et al.* Role of octreotide, scopolamine butylbromide and hydration in symptom control of patients with inoperable bowel obstruction and nasogastric tubes: a prospective randomized trial. *J Pain Symp Manage* 2000; **19**: 23–34.

97. Riley J, Fallon MT. Octreotide in terminal malignant obstruction of the gastrointestinal tract. *Eur J Palliat Care* 1994; **1** (1): 23–25.

98. Mercadante S. Scopolamine butylbromide plus octreotide in unresponsive bowel obstruction. *J Pain Symp Manage* 1998; **16**: 278–279.

99. Mulvenna PM, Regnard CFB. Subcutaneous ondansetron. *Lancet* 1992; **339**: 1059.

100. Currow DC, Coughlan M, Fardell B *et al.* Use of ondansetron in palliative medicine. *J Pain Symp Manage* 1997; **13** (5): 302–307.

101. Wilde MI, Markham A. Ondansetron: a review of its pharmacology and preliminary clinical findings in novel applications. *Drugs* 1996; **52** (5): 773–794.

102. Forman JK, Souney PF. Visual compatibility of midazolam hydrochloride with common preoperative injectable medications. *Am J Hosp Pharm* 1987; **44**: 2298–2299.

103. Parker WA. Physical compatibilities of preanaesthetic medications. *Can J Hosp Pharm* 1976; **29**: 91–92.

104. McIntyre P, Halifax, Canada. Personal communication.

105. Knapp AJ, Mauro VF, Alexander KS. Incompatibility of ketorolac tromethamine with selective postoperative drugs. *Am J Hosp Pharm* 1992; **49**: 2960–2962.

106. Formby F, Wollongong, Australia. Personal communication.

Chapter 3

Symptom Control with the Syringe Driver

Introduction

Palliative care patients often exhibit multiple pathology that can necessitate the use of numerous drug treatments. If the patient's condition deteriorates such that the oral route cannot be used, a continuous subcutaneous infusion (CSCI) via the syringe driver provides a simple and effective way to control symptoms. This chapter discusses how CSCIs can be used in the treatment of several distressing symptoms. Refer to Chapter 2 for drug information.

Pain

The dose of opioid to infuse depends upon previous requirements. A table of conversion factors is shown on p. 13. Unresolved somatic pain can be a cause of terminal agitation and must be anticipated, particularly since patients may have an exacerbation of pain at this time. Figures 6 and 7 provide simple algorithms of the points discussed below.

If the patient was previously taking a modified release (m/r) oral opioid, the CSCI should be started at the time the next dose was due. For practical purposes, a crossover period is generally not necessary. However, some practitioners recommend starting the driver 4 hours before the next m/r dose is due. In either case, to achieve or maintain adequate analgesia, a suitable subcutaneous bolus dose may be required.

If the patient is currently using a transdermal fentanyl patch, it is essential to continue with this. Breakthrough pain should be treated with equivalent 'rescue' doses of subcutaneous opioid. The total daily rescue medication is then given via a CSCI, in addition to the transdermal patch (Table 3).

Table 3 Determination of rescue doses of diamorphine for patients using a fentanyl patch.

Fentanyl Patch Strength	24–hour Diamorphine Dose	Rescue Dose
25microgram/hour	30 mg	5 mg
50microgram/hour	60 mg	10 mg
75microgram/hour	90 mg	15 mg
100microgram/hour	120 mg	20 mg

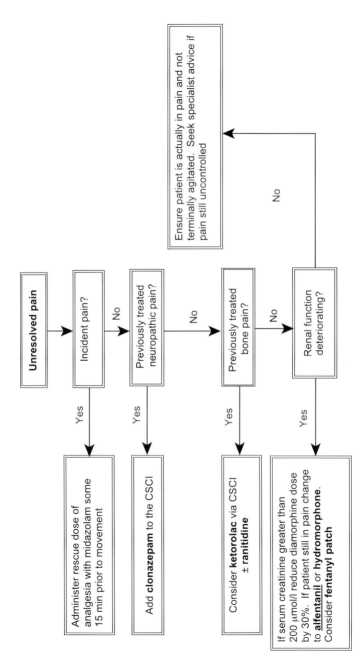

Fig. 7 Suggested treatment of unresolved pain.

Difficult cases

If the patient shows signs of *incident pain* (i.e. agitation or pain on movement), this is not an indication to increase the daily dose of analgesia. A suitable starting point for the treatment of incident pain is the administration of a rescue dose of opioid, coupled with a 5–10 mg subcutaneous dose of midazolam at least 15 minutes prior to movement. The use of midazolam here is to induce a state of amnesia, a useful effect of midazolam employed in surgery. In specialist centres, the use of alfentanil solely for incident pain may be considered, particularly as it has such a short duration of action. Since the patient experiencing incident pain is not in pain when at rest, any rescue dose of opioid given must *not* be included when calculating the new daily analgesia dose. This simple measure should prevent the rapid development of opioid toxicity. It would be sensible to prescribe separate opioid treatment on the prescription for incident pain to avoid this confusion.

Neuropathic pain is believed to be only partially responsive to opioid analgesia; hence the concurrent use of adjuvant analgesics. Unfortunately, most adjuvants cannot be given via CSCI. The exception is clonazepam, and some specialists may wish to consider the use of ketamine. Clonazepam should be considered (at an initial dose of 2–4 mg) if the patient is being treated for neuropathic pain, preferably before symptoms of pain become apparent. Note that clonazepam can be used to treat terminal agitation; the concurrent use of midazolam is not recommended. The use of ketamine should only be undertaken at specialist centres and will not be discussed here.

Renal failure can precipitate diamorphine/morphine toxicity due to the accumulation of the metabolite, morphine-6-glucuronide. Generally, if serum creatinine is greater than 200 μmol/l, or the patient clearly shows signs of opioid toxicity, the dose should be reduced by 30%. The rescue dose must also be amended. If the patient is uncomfortable after this reduction, the use of an alternative opioid should be considered. Alfentanil is suggested, although hydromorphone is another option. Fentanyl cannot be considered for use via the syringe driver because of volume constraints.

Musculoskeletal pain is also difficult to treat with opioids alone. Generally, this can be successfully controlled with the use of a nonsteroidal anti-inflammatory drug (NSAID) via a CSCI. **Ketorolac** is the recommended drug, although **diclofenac** has been used. These will more than likely necessitate the use of a second syringe driver and the dose of opioid must be reviewed. The practicalities of using a proton pump inhibitor must be considered.

Nausea and vomiting

One of the several indications for the use of a CSCI is uncontrolled nausea and vomiting. Nausea usually precedes vomiting and can be described as an unpleasant sensation associated with the urge to vomit. It causes gastric stasis, so an initial parenteral dose of an antiemetic will be necessary.

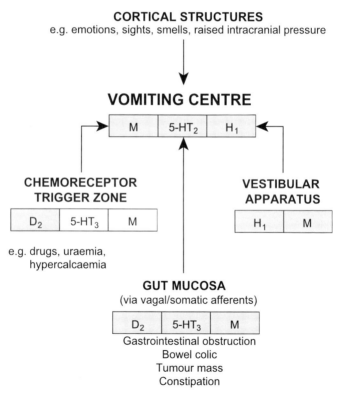

Fig. 8 Causes of nausea and vomiting. The shaded boxes represent prominent pharmacological targets.

It is important to have an understanding of the main neurotransmitters involved in the emetic process to ensure optimum pharmacological intervention (Fig. 8). The vomiting centre controls the complex act of vomiting and is located in the reticular formation of the lower medulla. Stimulation of the vomiting centre by impulses from the chemoreceptor trigger zone (CTZ), pharynx and gastrointestinal tract (via vagal and somatic afferents), vestibular apparatus and higher centres of the brain (e.g. visual cortex) results in emesis.

The CTZ is found in the area postrema and lies outside the blood–brain barrier. It is stimulated by emetic substances received through the blood as well as from the central nervous system. Dopamine (D_2), opioid (ν), serotonin ($5\text{-}HT_3$) and acetylcholine muscarinic (M) receptors have been located here, although the principal emetic pathway appears to be dopaminergic. The **nucleus tractus solitarius** is the main site for peripheral input from vagal and afferent neurons. D_2-, $5\text{-}HT_3$- and M-receptors are found here. Impulses from the **vestibular apparatus** pass through the vestibular nucleus (where histamine (H_1) and M-receptors are found) to the vomiting centre, via the cerebellum. Receptors found within the **vomiting centre** include $5\text{-}HT_2$, H_1 and M.

A thorough assessment and history is vital in order to identify the cause(s) of nausea and vomiting so as to enable the most suitable choice of antiemetic. Some of the common causes of nausea and vomiting encountered in palliative care are shown in Table 4.

Table 4 Possible causes of nausea and vomiting

- Drugs (eg opioids, cytotoxics, carbamazepine, digoxin, iron, NSAIDs)
- Gastroparesis
- Stress/anxiety
- Gastric ulceration
- Bowel obstruction
- Bowel colic
- Constipation
- Renal failure
- Hypercalcaemia
- Raised intracranial pressure

Antiemetics

The choice of antiemetic will depend on the cause(s) of nausea and vomiting. Most patients, however, have multiple and irreversible causes. Figure 9 illustrates the areas of the vomiting pathway where certain drugs act. Antiemetics may act at more than one type of receptor in producing their effect. For example, cyclizine may interact at both M- and H_1-receptors; metoclopramide acts at D_2-receptors and, at high doses, $5\text{-}HT_3$-receptors, an action that could contribute to its efficacy in controlling nausea and vomiting associated with cytotoxic agents. No currently available drug will antagonize *all* the receptor sites involved in the vomiting response. Neither is there a universal agent that will block the final common path-

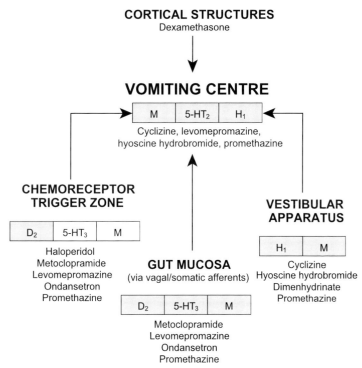

Fig. 9 The sites of action of selected antiemetics. The shaded boxes represent prominent pharmacological targets.

Table 5 Suggested treatments of nausea and vomiting using either a CSCI or subcutaneous injections.

Cause	First-line drug	Stat dose	Daily dose	Second-line drug[1]	Stat dose	Daily dose	Notes
Gastric stasis	Metoclopramide	10 mg (sc)	30–120 mg (CSCI)	–	–	–	Antimuscarinic drugs antagonize the effects of prokinetic drugs
Gastric irritation (e.g. drugs, tumour infiltration)	Metoclopramide	10 mg (sc)	30–120 mg (CSCI)	Levomepromazine or Ondansetron[2]	6.25 mg (sc) / 8 mg	6.25–25 mg (CSCI) / 24–32 mg (CSCI)	Consider oral proton pump inhibitor, if possible, or a CSCI of ranitidine 150–300 mg if NSAID induced
Total bowel obstruction with colic	Haloperidol or Promethazine[3] (used alone, no line drug)	1.5–5 mg (sc) / 25–50 mg (sc)	5–10 mg (CSCI) / 50–150 mg (CSCI)	Add cyclizine or Dimenhydrinate[4]	50 mg (sc) / 25–50 mg (sc)	100–150 mg (CSCI) / 50–200 mg (CSCI)	Ensure promethazine is not used with cyclizine or dimenhydrinate. In difficult cases, consider the use of dexamethasone 8–12 mg daily (sc) and review after 5 days
	Consider Hyoscine butylbromide or Glycopyrronium (for colic and may reduce volume of vomit)	20 mg (sc) / 400 micrograms (sc)	80–160 mg (CSCI) / 800–2400 micrograms (CSCI)	Levomepromazine	6.25 mg (sc)	6.25–25 mg (CSCI or sc stat)	Octreotide 300–600 micrograms daily (CSCI) with glyco-pyrronium may be beneficial if large-volume vomit

Table 5 Suggested treatments of nausea and vomiting using either a CSCI or subcutaneous injections (*contd.*).

Cause	First-line drug	Stat dose	Daily dose	Second-line drug[1]	Stat dose	Daily dose	Notes
Partial bowel obstruction without colic	Metoclopramide	10 mg (sc)	30–120 mg (CSCI)	Add dexamethasone	8–12 mg (sc)	8–12 mg (CSCI or sc stat)	Consider faecal softner (e.g. magnesium hydroxide 10 ml bd)
Chemoreceptor trigger zone (e.g. drugs, hypercalcaemia)	Haloperidol or Metoclopramide or Promethazine[3] (used alone)	1.5–5 mg (sc) / 50 mg (sc) / 25–50 mg (sc)	5–10 mg (CSCI) / 150 mg (CSCI) / 50–150 mg (CSCI)	Add cyclizine or Add dimenhydrinate[4] or Levomepromazine	50 mg (sc) / 25–50 mg (sc) / 6.25 mg (sc)	150 mg (CSCI) / 50–32 mg (CSCI) / 6.25–25 mg (CSCI or sc stat)	Ensure promethazine is used as the sole antiemetic
Raised intracranial pressure	Dexamethasone and either Cyclizine or Dimenhydrinate[4] or Promethazine	8–16 mg (sc) / 50 mg (sc) / 25–50 mg (sc) / 25–50 mg (sc)	8–16 mg (CSCI or sc stat) / 150 mg (CSCI) / 50–200 mg (CSCI) / 50–150 mg (CSCI)	Levomepromazine and Dexamethasone	6.25 mg (sc)	6.25–25 mg (CSCI or sc stat)	Do not administer dexamethasone and levomepromazine together via the same CSCI

1 Substitute the first-line drug with the second-line agent *unless* the table states otherwise.

2 Useful if problem is due to cellular damage with subsequent serotonin release, e.g. radiotherapy, renal failure.

3 Not generally considered in UK at present. Is used successfully in Australia.

4 Not available in the UK. Is a suitable alternative to cyclizine in Canada and USA.

way, the output from the vomiting centre. Consequently, a combination of agents may have a greater antiemetic action than a single drug. For resistant cases of nausea and vomiting, Table 5 should facilitate the choice of a suitable antiemetic. However, in general:

1 **Levomepromazine** 6.25–12.5 mg by subcutaneous injection at night is usually considered to be the most effective treatment in resistant cases.

2 If large volumes are being vomited, the use of antisecretory drugs such as **octreotide** 300 micrograms and **glycopyrronium** 1.2 mg can be considered.

3 The **5-HT$_3$ antagonists** are unlikely to be of benefit unless the cause of nausea/vomiting is due to damage of gastrointestinal enterochromaffin cells—i.e. recent radiotherapy/chemotherapy, or tumour infiltration.

Restlessness and agitation

General points

Terminal restlessness is defined as 'agitated delirium in a dying patient, frequently associated with impaired consciousness and myoclonic events'. Patients can suffer symptoms of agitation,

Table 6 Suggested causes of terminal agitation.

Drugs (e.g. opoids, antimuscarinic agents, carbamazepine, note that previously tolerated doses of drugs may become toxic as the disease progresses, or renal/liver deteriorates)
Pain
Brain tumour/metastases
Hypercalcaemia/hyp0onatraemia/hypoglycaemia
Renal failure/liver failure
Constipation
Urinary retention
Infection
Nicotine/alcohol withdrawal
Emotional distress (e.g. fear, anxiety)

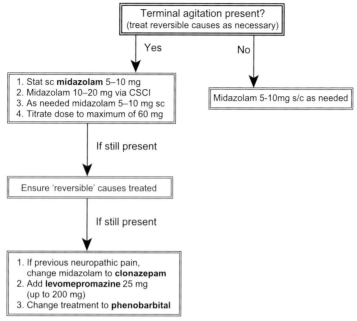

Fig. 10 The control of terminal agitation in the last 48 hours.

moaning/crying out, physical restlessness, myoclonic spasms or convulsions. Its presence can be distressing for both family and carer and may leave unpleasant, negative memories of an otherwise fairly peaceful dying process. The cause of terminal restlessness can be multifactorial; several causes are shown in Table 6. For patients close to death it is generally inappropriate to investigate and treat metabolic or infective causes (Fig. 10). However, other causes can be considered to be 'reversible' (underlined in Table 6) and these should be managed accordingly. If the patient is *not* close to death, *all* identified causes should be treated.

Management

1 Check to see if a 'reversible' cause as outlined above can be identified and treat accordingly, e.g. if the patient has suddenly stopped smoking, consider the use of a nicotine patch.

2 Ensure stat doses of **midazolam** are prescribed for breakthrough agitation/anxiety.

3 Begin titrating the dose of midazolam. Review requirements daily and add to a CSCI.

4 For more resistant forms of terminal restlessness, the following is suggested, in order:

(i) if previous neuropathic pain, change midazolam to **clonazepam** 4 mg (use 2 mg if less than 30 mg midazolam in 24 hours). The dose may need to be increased as necessary, up to 8 mg. Continue with midazolam for stat doses;

(ii) add **levomepromazine** 25 mg to the CSCI (check for compatibility). The dose can be increased as necessary (usually in 25–50 mg increments, depending on severity) up to a maximum of 200 mg. This drug is reserved as a second-line agent because of the potential for myoclonus. It is a useful adjunct to a benzodiazepine for uncontrolled agitation;

(iii) in the event that the above measures fail to control symptoms, change to **phenobarbital** 200 mg subcutaneously over 24 hours. This must be given via a separate driver. The dose can be increased if necessary to 600 mg.

Note

If midazolam and levomepromazine are unavailable, suitable alternatives include promethazine, hyoscine hydrobromide, haloperidol and phenobarbital. Note, however, that the former two drugs can cause paradoxical agitation

Respiratory tract secretions

Drugs will not be able to 'dry up' secretions already present, so it is important that treatment is initiated as soon as symptoms appear (Fig. 11). The 'death rattle' is more disturbing for relatives and carers than the patient, who is usually semiconscious.

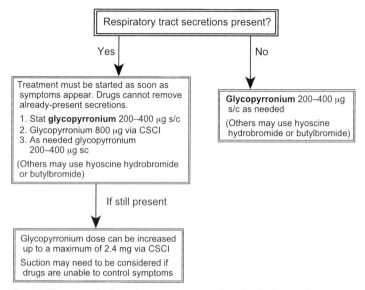

Fig. 11 The control of respiratory tract secretions in the last 48 hours.

In addition to patient positioning, the pharmacological options via CSCI over 24 hours include **glycopyrronium** 0.6–2.4 mg, **hyoscine hydrobromide** 1.2–2.4 mg and **hyoscine hydrobromide** 20–180 mg. Glycopyrronium is generally preferred due to the perceived pharmacological benefits and cost effectiveness. Note, however, that there is no evidence to support the superiority of either drug. Stat doses must be prescribed for breakthrough secretions. Some centres use **hyoscine butylbromide,** a cheaper drug than glycopyrronium, but possibly not as effective.

The volume of glycopyrronium injection is likely to be the main problem encountered with the treatment of this condition. The maximum 2.4 mg dose of glycopyrronium equates to 12 ml of liquid. The Graseby MS26 can infuse a maximum of 20–25 ml (using a 35 ml syringe). It is possible that the total volume to be infused will exceed this amount. In such cases, a 12-hourly infusion rate will be needed.

Chapter 4

Compatibility Data Tables

Compatibility data tables

Two drugs

Alfentanil (A) and Clonazepam (B)

Summary: No problems with physical stability encountered

Drug	Dose in syringe (mg)	Volume in syringe (ml)	Concentration (mg/ml)	Diluent	Outcome	Data type
A	80	20	4.00	Water for injections	Physically stable over 24 h	Laboratory
B	4		0.20			

Alfentanil (A) and Cyclizine (B)

Summary: Problems with physical compatibility are likely as concentrations of either drug increase (compare diamorphine/cyclizine)

Drug	Dose in syringe (mg)	Volume in syringe (ml)	Concentration (mg/ml)	Diluent	Outcome	Data type
A	2	17	0.12	Water for injections	Physically stable over 24 h	Clinical observation
B	150		8.82			
A	4	17	0.24	Water for injections	Physically stable over 24 h	Clinical observation
B	150		8.82			
A	85	20	4.25	Water for injections	Incompatible	Laboratory
B	150		7.50			

Alfentanil (A) and Dexamethasone (B)

Summary: No problems with physical stability encountered. Dexamethasone is usually given as a subcutaneous bolus injection

Drug	Dose in syringe (mg)	Volume in syringe (ml)	Concentration (mg/ml)	Diluent	Outcome	Data type
A	80	20	4.00	Water for injections	Physically stable over 24 h	Laboratory
B	16		0.80			

Alfentanil (A) and **Glycopyrronium (B)**

Summary: No problems with physical stability encountered

Drug	Dose in syringe (mg)	Volume in syringe (ml)	Concentration (mg/ml)	Diluent	Outcome	Data type
A	60	20	3.00	Water for injections	Physically stable over 24 h	Laboratory
B	1.6		0.08			

Alfentanil (A) and **Haloperidol (B)**

Summary: No problems with physical stability encountered

Drug	Dose in syringe (mg)	Volume in syringe (ml)	Concentration (mg/ml)	Diluent	Outcome	Data type
A	85	20	4.25	Water for injections	Physically stable over 24 h	Laboratory
B	15		0.75			

Alfentanil (A) and **Hyosine Butylbromide (B)**

Summary: No problems with physical stability encountered

Drug	Dose in syringe (mg)	Volume in syringe (ml)	Concentration (mg/ml)	Diluent	Outcome	Data type
A	70	20	3.50	Water for injections	Physically stable over 24 h	Laboratory
B	120		6.00			

Alfentanil (A) and **Levomepromazine (B)**

Summary: No problems with physical stability encountered

Drug	Dose in syringe (mg)	Volume in syringe (ml)	Concentration (mg/ml)	Diluent	Outcome	Data type
A	3	8	0.38	Water for injections	Physically stable over 24 h	Clinical observation
B	12.5		1.56			
A	90	20	4.50	Water for injections	Physically stable over 24 h	Laboratory
B	50		2.50			

Alfentanil (A) and **Metoclopramide (B)**

Summary: No problems with physical stability encountered

Drug	Dose in syringe (mg)	Volume in syringe (ml)	Concentration (mg/ml)	Diluent	Outcome	Data type
A	60	20	3.00	Water for injections	Physically stable over 24 h	Laboratory
B	40		2.00			

Alfentanil (A) and **Midazolam (B)**

Summary: No problems with physical stability encountered

Drug	Dose in syringe (mg)	Volume in syringe (ml)	Concentration (mg/ml)	Diluent	Outcome	Data type
A	3	10	0.30	Water for injections	Physically stable over 24 h	Clinical observation
B	30		3.00			
A	60	20	3.00	Water for injections	Physically stable over 24 h	Laboratory
B	40		2.00			

Diamorphine (A) and Cyclizine (B)

Summary: Physically compatible, although crystallisation may occur if the concentration of either drug is greater than 10 mg/ml. See Chapter 2 for more details.

Drug	Dose in syringe (mg)	Volume in syringe (ml)	Concentration (mg/ml)	Diluent	Outcome	Data type
A	20	17	1.18	Water for injections	Physically stable over 24 h	Clinical observation
B	150		8.82			
A	40	17	2.35	Water for injections	Physically stable over 24 h	Clinical observation
B	150		8.82			
A	100	17	5.88	Water for injections	Physically stable over 24 h	Clinical observation
B	150		8.82			
A	130	17	7.65	Water for injections	Physically stable over 24 h	Clinical observation
B	150		8.82			
A	450	17	26.47	Water for injections	Physically stable over 24 h	Clinical observation
B	150		8.82			
A	550	17	32.35	Water for injections	Physically stable over 24 h	Clinical observation
B	150		8.82			
A	840	9.5	88.42	Water for injections	Incompatible see summary above	Clinical observation
B	150		15.79			

Diamorphine (A) and Dexamethasone (B)

Summary: No problems with physical stability encountered, although precipitation/turbidity may occur as dexamethasone dose increases. Note that diamorphine degradation increases as the pH increases. Dexamethasone is usually given as a subcutaneous bolus injection

Drug	Dose in syringe (mg)	Volume in syringe (ml)	Concentration (mg/ml)	Diluent	Outcome	Data type
A	15	17	0.88	Water for injections	Physically stable over 24 h	Clinical observation
B	16		0.94			
A	50	16	3.13	Water for injections	Physically stable over 24 h	Clinical observation
B	12		0.75			
A	70	17	4.12	Water for injections	Physically stable over 24 h	Clinical observation
B	8		0.47			

Diamorphine (A) and Haloperidol (B)

Summary: No problems with physical stability encountered

Drug	Dose in syringe (mg)	Volume in syringe (ml)	Concentration (mg/ml)	Diluent	Outcome	Data type
A	30	17	1.76	Water for injections	Physically stable over 24 h	Clinical observation
B	5		0.29			
A	45	17	2.65	Water for injections	Physically stable over 24 h	Clinical observation
B	0		0.59			
A	80	17	4.71	Water for injections	Physically stable over 24 h	Clinical observation
B	15		0.88			
A	300	15	20.00	Water for injections	Physically stable over 24 h	Clinical observation
B	10		0.67			
A	430	15	28.67	Water for injections	Physically stable over 24 h	Clinical observation
B	15		1.00			
A	500	17	29.41	Water for injections	Physically stable over 24 h	Clinical observation
B	10		0.59			

Diamorphine (A) and Hyoscine Butylbromide (B)

Summary: No problems with physical stability encountered

Drug	Dose in syringe (mg)	Volume in syringe (ml)	Concentration (mg/ml)	Diluent	Outcome	Data type
A	20	17	1.18	Water for injections	Physically stable over 24 h	Clinical observation
B	60		3.53			
A	30	17	1.76	Water for injections	Physically stable over 24 h	Laboratory
B	80		4.71			
A	70	17	4.12	Water for injections	Physically stable over 24 h	Laboratory
B	80		4.71			
A	100	17	5.88	Water for injections	Physically stable over 24 h	Clinical observation
B	120		7.06			

Diamorphine (A) and Ketorolac (B)

Summary: No problems with physical stability encountered. However, degradation of diamorphine can occur at high pH (see drug information Chapter 2)

Drug	Dose in syringe (mg)	Volume in syringe (ml)	Concentration (mg/ml)	Diluent	Outcome	Data type
A	50	8.5	5.88	Sodium chloride 0.9%	Physically stable over 24 h	Clinical observation
B	90		10.59			

Diamorphine (A) and Levomepromazine (B)

Summary: No problems with physical stability encountered. To avoid irritation at the site of infusion, levomepromazine may be given as a bolus subcutaneous injection at doses below 50 mg (= 2 ml)

Drug	Dose in syringe (mg)	Volume in syringe (ml)	Concentration (mg/ml)	Diluent	Outcome	Data type
A	50	17	2.94	Water for injections	Physically stable over 24 h	Clinical observation
B	18.75		1.10			
A	150	17	8.82	Water for injections	Physically stable over 24 h	Clinical observation
B	25		1.47			
A	80	9	8.89	Water for injections	Physically stable over 24 h	Clinical observation
B	37.5		4.17			
A	200	17	11.76	Water for injections	Physically stable over 24 h	Clinical observation
B	25		1.47			
A	200	17	11.76	Water for injections	Physically stable over 24 h	Clinical observation
B	50		2.94			
A	180	10	18.00	Water for injections	Physically stable over 24 h	Clinical observation
B	25		2.50			

Diamorphine (A) and Metoclopramide (B)

Summary: No problems with physical stability encountered

Drug	Dose in syringe (mg)	Volume in syringe (ml)	Concentration (mg/ml)	Diluent	Outcome	Data type
A	40	17	2.35	Water for injections	Physically stable over 24 h	Clinical observation
B	30		1.76			
A	50	17	2.94	Water for injections	Physically stable over 24 h	Clinical observation
B	40		2.35			
A	150	17	8.82	Water for injections	Physically stable over 24 h	Clinical observation
B	60		3.53			
A	350	10	35.00	Water for injections	Physically stable over 24 h	Clinical observation
B	30		3.00			

Diamorphine (A) and Midazolam (B)

Summary: No problems with physical stability encountered

Drug	Dose in syringe (mg)	Volume in syringe (ml)	Concentration (mg/ml)	Diluent	Outcome	Data type
A	10	17	0.59	Water for injections	Physically stable over 24 h	Clinical observation
B	10		0.59			
A	50	17	2.94	Water for injections	Physically stable over 24 h	Clinical observation
B	20		1.18			
A	180	17	10.59	Water for injections	Physically stable over 24 h	Clinical observation
B	40		2.35			
A	320	15	21.33	Water for injections	Physically stable over 24 h	Clinical observation
B	60		4.00			
A	450	17	26.47	Water for injections	Physically stable over 24 h	Clinical observation
B	25		1.47			
A	1400	17	82.35	Water for injections	Physically stable over 24 h	Clinical observation
B	30		1.76			
A	2300	15	153.3	Water for injections	Physically stable over 24 h	Clinical observation
B	30		2.00			

Diamorphine (A) and Octreotide (B)

Summary: No problems with physical stability encountered

Drug	Dose in syringe (mg)	Volume in syringe (ml)	Concentration (mg/ml)	Diluent	Outcome	Data type
A	120	17	7.06	Water for injections	Physically stable over 24 h	Clinical observation
B	0.6		0.04			
A	280	17	16.47	Water for injections	Physically stable over 24 h	Clinical observation
B	0.6		0.04			

Diamorphine (A) and Ondansetron (B)

Summary: No problems with physical stability encountered

Drug	Dose in syringe (mg)	Volume in syringe (ml)	Concentration (mg/ml)	Diluent	Outcome	Data type
A	720	17	40.00	Water for injections	Physically stable over 24 h	Clinical observation
B	24		1.60			

Dihydrocodeine (A) and Cyclizine (B)

Summary: No problems with physical stability encountered

Drug	Dose in syringe (mg)	Volume in syringe (ml)	Concentration (mg/ml)	Diluent	Outcome	Data type
A	150	20	7.50	Water for injections	Physically stable over 24 h	Laboratory
B	150		7.50			

Dihydrocodeine (A) and Dexamethasone (B)

Summary: No problems with physical stability encountered

Drug	Dose in syringe (mg)	Volume in syringe (ml)	Concentration (mg/ml)	Diluent	Outcome	Data type
A	150	20	7.50	Water for injections	Physically stable over 24 h	Laboratory
B	16		0.80			

Dihydrocodeine (A) and Haloperidol (B)

Summary: No problems with physical stability encountered

Drug	Dose in syringe (mg)	Volume in syringe (ml)	Concentration (mg/ml)	Diluent	Outcome	Data type
A	150	20	7.50	Water for injections	Physically stable over 24 h	Laboratory
B	15		0.75			

Dihydrocodeine (A) and Levomepromazine (B)

Summary: No problems with physical stability encountered

Drug	Dose in syringe (mg)	Volume in syringe (ml)	Concentration (mg/ml)	Diluent	Outcome	Data type
A	150	20	7.50	Water for injections	Physically stable over 24 h	Laboratory
B	50		2.50			

Methadone (A) and Clonazepam (B)

Summary: No problems with physical stability encountered

Drug	Dose in syringe (mg)	Volume in syringe (ml)	Concentration (mg/ml)	Diluent	Outcome	Data type
A	60	17	3.53	Sodium chloride 0.9%	Physically stable over 24 h	Clinical observation
B	2		0.12			

Methadone (A) and Midazolam (B)

Summary: No problems with physical stability encountered

Drug	Dose in syringe (mg)	Volume in syringe (ml)	Concentration (mg/ml)	Diluent	Outcome	Data type
A	25	16	1.56	Sodium chloride 0.9%	Physically stable over 24 h	Clinical observation
B	20		1.25			

Tramadol (A) and Haloperidol (B)

Summary: No problems with physical stability encountered

Drug	Dose in syringe (mg)	Volume in syringe (ml)	Concentration (mg/ml)	Diluent	Outcome	Data type
A	200	17	11.76	Water for injections	Physically stable over 24 h	Clinical observation
B	10		0.59			
A	300	17	17.65	Water for injections	Physically stable over 24 h	Clinical observation
B	5		0.29			

Tramadol (A) and Promethazine (B)

Summary: No problems with physical stability encountered

Drug	Dose in syringe (mg)	Volume in syringe (ml)	Concentration (mg/ml)	Diluent	Outcome	Data type
A	200	18	11.11	Water for injections	Physically stable over 24 h	Laboratory
B	100		5.56			

Clonazepam (A) and Dexamethasone (B)

Summary: No problems with physical stability encountered. Dexamethasone is usually given as a subcutaneous bolus injection

Drug	Dose in syringe (mg)	Volume in syringe (ml)	Concentration (mg/ml)	Diluent	Outcome	Data type
A	2	17	0.12	Water for injections	Physically stable over 24 h	Clinical observation
B	16		0.94			
A	6	17	0.35	Water for injections	Physically stable over 24 h	Clinical observation
B	6		0.35			

Clonazepam (A) and Glycopyrronium (B)

Summary: No problems with physical stability encountered

Drug	Dose in syringe (mg)	Volume in syringe (ml)	Concentration (mg/ml)	Diluent	Outcome	Data type
A	4	17	0.24	Water for injections	Physically stable over 24 h	Clinical observation
B	1.2		0.07			

Cyclizine (A) and Metoclopramide (B)

Summary: Crystallization may occur as dose of metoclopramide increases relative to cyclizine. This is **not** a sensible combination of anti-emetics, since the prokinetic action of metoclopramide is inhibited by cyclizine. Higher doses of metoclopramide will be required to overcome this. However, use of this combination is acceptable if metoclopramide is used for its central dopamine antagonist properties

Drug	Dose in syringe (mg)	Volume in syringe (ml)	Concentration (mg/ml)	Diluent	Outcome	Data type
A	150	17	8.82	Water for injections	Physically stable over 24 h	Clinical observation
B	30		1.76			
A	150	10	15.00	Water for injections	Mixed results. See summary.	Clinical observation
B	60		6.00			

Dexamethasone (A) and Haloperidol (B)

Summary: Physically incompatible; precipitated immediately. Note if diamorphine is included, the combination appears to be physically stable (see below). Dexamethasone is usually given as a subcutaneous bolus injection

Drug	Dose in syringe (mg)	Volume in syringe (ml)	Concentration (mg/ml)	Diluent	Outcome	Data type
A	12	20	0.60	Water for injections	Incompatible	Laboratory
B	5		0.25			

Dexamethasone (A) and Levomepromazine (B)

Summary: Combination may be incompatible as the dose of dexamethasone increases; higher concentrations will precipitate immediately. Dexamethasone is usually given as a subcutaneous bolus injection. To avoid irritation at the infusion site, levomepromazine may be given as a bolus subcutaneous injection at doses below 50 mg (= 2 ml).

Drug	Dose in syringe (mg)	Volume in syringe (ml)	Concentration (mg/ml)	Diluent	Outcome	Data type
A	1	9	0.11	Water for injections	Physically stable over 24 h	Clinical observation
B	25		2.78			
A	8	15	0.53	Water for injections	**Incompatible**	Clinical observation
B	50		3.33			

Dexamethasone (A) and Midazolam (B)

Summary: No problems with physical stability encountered, although precipitation/turbidity may occur as doses increase (pH effect). Dexamethasone is usually given as a subcutaneous bolus injection

Drug	Dose in syringe (mg)	Volume in syringe (ml)	Concentration (mg/ml)	Diluent	Outcome	Data type
A	8	15	0.53	Water for injections	Physically stable over 24 h	Clinical observation
B	35		2.33			

Glycopyrronium (A) and Ranitidine (B)

Summary: No problems with physical stability encountered

Drug	Dose in syringe (mg)	Volume in syringe (ml)	Concentration (mg/ml)	Diluent	Outcome	Data type
A	0.6	17	0.04	Water for injections	Physically stable over 24 h	Clinical observation
B	150		8.82			

Haloperidol (A) and Hyoscine Butylbromide (B)

Summary: No problems with physical stability encountered

Drug	Dose in syringe (mg)	Volume in syringe (ml)	Concentration (mg/ml)	Diluent	Outcome	Data type
A	5	15	0.33	Water for injections	Physically stable over 24 h	Clinical observation
B	80		5.33			

Haloperidol (A) and Ketamine (B)

Summary: No problems with physical stability encountered

Drug	Dose in syringe (mg)	Volume in syringe (ml)	Concentration (mg/ml)	Diluent	Outcome	Data type
A	10	8	1.25	Sodium chloride 0.9%	Physically stable over 24 h	Clinical observation
B	150		18.75			

Ketamine (A) and Midazolam (B)

Summary: No problems with physical stability encountered

Drug	Dose in syringe (mg)	Volume in syringe (ml)	Concentration (mg/ml)	Diluent	Outcome	Data type
A	300	9.5	31.58	Sodium chloride 0.9%	Physically stable over 24 h	Clinical observation
B	20		2.11			

Ketorolac (A) and Ranitidine (B)

Summary: No problems with physical stability encountered.

Drug	Dose in syringe (mg)	Volume in syringe (ml)	Concentration (mg/ml)	Diluent	Outcome	Data type
A	90	20	4.50	Sodium chloride 0.9%	Physically stable over 24 h	Laboratory
B	150		7.50			

Levomepromazine (A) and Octreotide (B)

Summary: No problems with physical stability encountered. To avoid irritation at the site of the infusion, levomepromazine may be given as a bolus subcutaneous injection at doses below 50 mg (= 2 ml).

Drug	Dose in syringe (mg)	Volume in syringe (ml)	Concentration (mg/ml)	Diluent	Outcome	Data type
A	50	17	2.94	Water for injections	Physically stable over 24 h	Clinical observation
B	0.6		0.04			

Metoclopramide (A) and Octreotide (B)

Summary: No problems with physical stability encountered

Drug	Dose in syringe (mg)	Volume in syringe (ml)	Concentration (mg/ml)	Diluent	Outcome	Data type
A	60	17	3.53	Water for injections	Physically stable over 24 h	Clinical observation
B	0.6		0.04			

Drug A	B	C	page
Alfentanil	Clonazepam	Glycopyrronium	92
Alfentanil	Clonazepam	Haloperidol	92
Alfentanil	Clonazepam	Hyoscine Hydrobromide	92
Alfentanil	Cyclizine	Midazolam	93
Alfentanil	Haloperidol	Midazolam	93
Alfentanil	Hyoscine Butylbromide	Levomepromazine	93
Alfentanil	Metoclopramide	Midazolam	94
Diamorphine	Clonazepam	Cyclizine	94
Diamorphine	Clonazepam	Dexamethasone	95
Diamorphine	Clonazepam	Glycopyrronium	95
Diamorphine	Clonazepam	Haloperidol	95
Diamorphine	Clonazepam	Hyoscine Butylbromide	96
Diamorphine	Clonazepam	Levomepromazine	96
Diamorphine	Cyclizine	Dexamethasone	97
Diamorphine	Cyclizine	Haloperidol	98
Diamorphine	Cyclizine	Hyoscine Butylbromide	99
Diamorphine	Cyclizine	Hyoscine Hydrobromide	99
Diamorphine	Cyclizine	Levomepromazine	99
Diamorphine	Cyclizine	Metoclopramide	100
Diamorphine	Cyclizine	Midazolam	101
Diamorphine	Dexamethasone	Haloperidol	102
Diamorphine	Dexamethasone	Hyoscine Hydrobromide	102
Diamorphine	Dexamethasone	Levomepromazine	103
Diamorphine	Dexamethasone	Metoclopramide	103
Diamorphine	Dexamethasone	Midazolam	104
Diamorphine	Dexamethasone	Ondansetron	104
Diamorphine	Glycopyrronium	Levomepromazine	104
Diamorphine	Glycopyrronium	Midazolam	105
Diamorphine	Haloperidol	Hyoscine Butylbromide	105
Diamorphine	Haloperidol	Levomepromazine	106
Diamorphine	Haloperidol	Metoclopramide	106
Diamorphine	Haloperidol	Midazolam	107
Diamorphine	Hyoscine Butylbromide	Levomepromazine	108

Compatibility data tables

Three drugs

Alfentanil (A), Clonazepam (B) and Glycopyrronium (C)

Summary: No problems with physical stability encountered

Drug	Dose in syringe (mg)	Volume in syringe (ml)	Concentration (mg/ml)	Diluent	Outcome	Data type
A	10		0.67			
B	4	15	0.27	Water for injections	Physically stable over 24 h	Clinical observation
C	1.8		0.12			

Alfentanil (A), Clonazepam (B) and Haloperidol (C)

Summary: No problems with physical stability encountered

Drug	Dose in syringe (mg)	Volume in syringe (ml)	Concentration (mg/ml)	Diluent	Outcome	Data type
A	2		0.13			
B	4	16	0.25	Water for injections	Physically stable over 24 h	Clinical observation
C	5		0.31			

Alfentanil (A), Clonazepam (B) and Hyoscine Hydrobromide (C)

Summary: No problems with physical stability encountered

Drug	Dose in syringe (mg)	Volume in syringe (ml)	Concentration (mg/ml)	Diluent	Outcome	Data type
A	10		0.67			
B	2	15	0.13	Water for injections	Physically stable over 24 h	Clinical observation
C	1.8		0.12			

Alfentanil (A), Cyclizine (B) and Midazolam (C)

Summary: No problems with physical stability encountered. Crystallisation may occur as concentrations increase.

Drug	Dose in syringe (mg)	Volume in syringe (ml)	Concentration (mg/ml)	Diluent	Outcome	Data type
A	3		0.18	Water for injections	Physically stable over 24 h	Clinical observation
B	150	17	8.82			
C	20		1.18			
A	55		3.06	Water for injections	Physically stable over 24 h	Clinical observation
B	75	18	4.17			
C	20		1.11			
A	75		3.00	Water for injections	Physically stable over 24 h	Clinical observation
B	150	25	6.00			
C	30		1.20			

Alfentanil (A), Haloperidol (B) and Midazolam (C)

Summary: No problems with physical stability encountered

Drug	Dose in syringe (mg)	Volume in syringe (ml)	Concentration (mg/ml)	Diluent	Outcome	Data type
A	14.5		1.12	Water for injections	Physically stable over 24 h	Clinical observation
B	5	13	0.38			
C	30		2.31			

Alfentanil (A), Hyoscine Butylbromide (B) and Levomepromazine (C)

Summary: No problems with physical stability encountered. To reduce irritation at the site of infusion, levomepromazine may be given as a subcutaneous bolus injection at doses below 50 mg (= 2 ml)

Drug	Dose in syringe (mg)	Volume in syringe (ml)	Concentration (mg/ml)	Diluent	Outcome	Data type
A	6		0.40	Water for injections	Physically stable over 24 h	Clinical observation
B	100	15	6.67			
C	12.5		0.83			

Alfentanil (A), Metoclopramide (B) and **Midazolam (C)**

Summary: No problems with physical stability encountered

Drug	Dose in syringe (mg)	Volume in syringe (ml)	Concentration (mg/ml)	Diluent	Outcome	Data type
A	3		0.20	Water for injections	Physically stable over 24 h	Clinical observation
B	30	15	2.00			
C	40		2.67			
A	6		0.35	Water for injections	Physically stable over 24 h	Clinical observation
B	60	17	3.53			
C	10		0.59			
A	14		1.00	Water for injections	Physically stable over 24 h	Clinical observation
B	30	14	2.14			
C	20		1.43			

Diamorphine (A), Clonazepam (B) and **Cyclizine (C)**

Summary: No problems with physical stability encountered. Crystallisation may occur as concentrations increase

Drug	Dose in syringe (mg)	Volume in syringe (ml)	Concentration (mg/ml)	Diluent	Outcome	Data type
A	100		6.67	Water for injections	Physically stable over 24 h	Clinical observation
B	4	15	0.27			
C	150		10.00			
A	520		30.59	Water for injections	Physically stable over 24 h	Clinical observation
B	6	17	0.35			
C	150		8.82			

Diamorphine (A), Clonazepam (B)
and **Dexamethasone (C)**

Summary: No problems with physical stability encountered. Dexamethasone is usually given as a subcutaneous bolus injection

Drug	Dose in syringe (mg)	Volume in syringe (ml)	Concentration (mg/ml)	Diluent	Outcome	Data type
A	20		1.18	Water for injections	Physically stable over 24 h	Clinical observation
B	4	17	0.24			
C	8		0.47			

Diamorphine (A), Clonazepam (B)
and **Glycopyrronium (C)**

Summary: No problems with physical stability encountered

Drug	Dose in syringe (mg)	Volume in syringe (ml)	Concentration (mg/ml)	Diluent	Outcome	Data type
A	60		3.53	Water for injections	Physically stable over 24 h	Clinical observation
B	2	17	0.12			
C	0.6		0.04			

Diamorphine (A), Clonazepam (B)
and **Haloperidol (C)**

Summary: No problems with physical stability encountered

Drug	Dose in syringe (mg)	Volume in syringe (ml)	Concentration (mg/ml)	Diluent	Outcome	Data type
A	20		2.22	Water for injections	Physically stable over 24 h	Clinical observation
B	1	9	0.11			
C	5		0.56			
A	30		1.76	Water for injections	Physically stable over 24 h	Clinical observation
B	8	17	0.47			
C	5		0.29			

Diamorphine (A), Clonazepam (B) and **Hyoscine Butylbromide (C)**

Summary: No problems with physical stability encountered

Drug	Dose in syringe (mg)	Volume in syringe (ml)	Concentration (mg/ml)	Diluent	Outcome	Data type
A	1800		112.5	Water for injections	Physically stable over 24 h	Clinical observation
B	3	16	0.19			
C	120		7.50			

Diamorphine (A), Clonazepam (B) and **Levomepromazine (C)**

Summary: No problems with physical stability encountered. To reduce irritation at the site of infusion, levomepromazine may be given as a subcutaneous bolus injection at doses below 50 mg (= 2 ml)

Drug	Dose in syringe (mg)	Volume in syringe (ml)	Concentration (mg/ml)	Diluent	Outcome	Data type
A	600		35.29	Water for injections	Physically stable over 24 h	Clinical observation
B	3	17	0.18			
C	18.75		1.10			
A	950		55.88	Water for injections	Physically stable over 24 h	Clinical observation
B	2	17	0.12			
C	25		1.47			

Diamorphine (A), Cyclizine (B) and **Dexamethasone (C)**

Summary: No problems with physical stability encountered, although precipitation/turbidity may occur as doses increase. Dexamethasone is usually given as a subcutaneous bolus injection

Drug	Dose in syringe (mg)	Volume in syringe (ml)	Concentration (mg/ml)	Diluent	Outcome	Data type
A	80		4.71	Water for injections	Physically stable over 24 h	Clinical observation
B	150	17	8.82			
C	6		0.35			
A	100		5.88	Water for injections	Physically stable over 24 h	Clinical observation
B	150	17	8.82			
C	12		0.71			
A	140		8.24	Water for injections	Physically stable over 24 h	Clinical observation
B	150	17	8.82			
C	8		0.47			
A	250		16.67	Water for injections	Physically stable over 24 h	Clinical observation
B	150	17	10.00			
C	6		0.40			

Diamorphine (A), Cyclizine (B) and Haloperidol (C)

Summary: No problems with physical stability encountered. Crystallisation may occur as concentrations increase.

Drug	Dose in syringe (mg)	Volume in syringe (ml)	Concentration (mg/ml)	Diluent	Outcome	Data type
A	15		0.88			
B	150	17	8.82	Water for injections	Physically stable over 24 h	Clinical observation
C	5		0.29			
A	20		1.18			
B	150	17	8.82	Water for injections	Physically stable over 24 h	Clinical observation
C	15		0.88			
A	50		2.94			
B	150	17	8.82	Water for injections	Physically stable over 24 h	Clinical observation
C	5		0.29			
A	60		4.00			
B	150	15	10.00	Water for injections	Physically stable over 24 h	Clinical observation
C	10		0.67			
A	60		6.00			
B	150	10	15.00	Water for injections	Physically stable over 24 h	Clinical observation
C	10		1.00			
A	150		9.38			
B	150	16	9.38	Water for injections	Physically stable over 24 h	Clinical observation
C	10		0.63			
A	800		57.14			
B	150	14	10.71	Water for injections	Physically stable over 24 h	Clinical observation
C	10		0.71			

Diamorphine (A), Cyclizine (B) and **Hyoscine Butylbromide (C)**

Summary: Cyclizine may crystallize with hyoscine butylbromide and/or diamorphine. If an anticholinergic drug is required, glyco-pyrronium is an acceptable alternative

Drug	Dose in syringe (mg)	Volume in syringe (ml)	Concentration (mg/ml)	Diluent	Outcome	Data type
A	35		2.19			
B	150	16	9.38	Water for injections	Incompatible	Clinical observation
C	80		5.00			
A	160		10.67			
B	150	15	10.00	Water for injections	Incompatible	Clinical observation
C	40		2.67			

Diamorphine (A), Cyclizine (B) and **Hyoscine Hydrobromide (C)**

Summary: No problems with physical stability encountered. Crystallisation may occur as concentrations increase.

Drug	Dose in syringe (mg)	Volume in syringe (ml)	Concentration (mg/ml)	Diluent	Outcome	Data type
A	60		3.53			
B	150	17	8.82	Water for injections	Physically stable over 24 h	Clinical observation
C	1.6		0.09			

Diamorphine (A), Cyclizine (B) and **Levomepromazine (C)**

Summary: No problems with physical stability encountered. Crystalli-sation may occur as concentrations increase. To reduce irritation at the site of infusion, levomepromazine may be given as a subcutaneous bolus injection at doses below 50 mg (= 2 ml)

Drug	Dose in syringe (mg)	Volume in syringe (ml)	Concentration (mg/ml)	Diluent	Outcome	Data type
A	180		10.59			
B	150	17	8.82	Water for injections	Physically stable over 24 h	Clinical observation
C	25		1.47			
A	540		31.76			
B	150	17	8.82	Water for injections	Physically stable over 24 h	Clinical observation
C	100		5.88			

Diamorphine (A), Cyclizine (B) and **Metoclopramide (C)**

Summary: Crystallization may occur as concentrations increase. This is **not** a sensible combination of antiemetics, since the prokinetic action of metoclopramide is inhibited by cyclizine. Higher doses of metoclopramide will be required to overcome this. However, use of this combination is acceptable if metoclopramide is used for its central dopamine antagonist properties

Drug	Dose in syringe (mg)	Volume in syringe (ml)	Concentration (mg/ml)	Diluent	Outcome	Data type
A	25		1.47			
B	150	17	8.82	Water for injections	Incompatible	Clinical observation
C	40		2.35			
A	40		2.35			
B	200	17	11.76	Water for injections	Incompatible	Clinical observation
C	60		3.53			
A	120		7.06			
B	75	17	4.41	Water for injections	Physically stable over 24 h	Clinical observation
C	30		1.76			

Diamorphine (A), Cyclizine (B) and Midazolam (C)

Summary: No problems with physical stability encountered. Crystallisation may occur as concentrations increase.

Drug	Dose in syringe (mg)	Volume in syringe (ml)	Concentration (mg/ml)	Diluent	Outcome	Data type
A	35		2.06	Water for injections	Physically stable over 24 h	Clinical observation
B	150	17	8.82			
C	20		1.18			
A	40		2.35	Water for injections	Physically stable over 24 h	Clinical observation
B	150	17	8.82			
C	30		1.76			
A	60		3.33	Water for injections	Physically stable over 24 h	Clinical observation
B	150	18	8.33			
C	30		1.67			
A	70		4.12	Water for injections	Physically stable over 24 h	Clinical observation
B	150	17	8.82			
C	40		2.35			
A	160		9.41	Water for injections	Physically stable over 24 h	Clinical observation
B	150	17	8.82			
C	30		1.76			
A	320		20.00	Water for injections	Physically stable over 24 h	Clinical observation
B	150	16	9.38			
C	30		1.18			
A	630		37.06	Water for injections	Physically stable over 24 h	Clinical observation
B	150	17	8.82			
C	40		2.35			

Diamorphine (A), Dexamethasone (B) and **Haloperidol (C)**

Summary: No problems with physical stability encountered, although precipitation/turbidity may occur as doses increase. Note that the mixture of dexamethasone and haloperidol alone has been shown to be incompatible. It is usual to give dexamethasone as a subcutaneous bolus injection

Drug	Dose in syringe (mg)	Volume in syringe (ml)	Concentration (mg/ml)	Diluent	Outcome	Data type
A	50		2.94			
B	6	17	0.35	Water for injections	Physically stable over 24 h	Clinical observation
C	5		0.29			
A	60		3.53			
B	16	17	0.94	Water for injections	Physically stable over 24 h	Clinical observation
C	5		0.29			
A	100		5.88			
B	8	17	0.47	Water for injections	Physically stable over 24 h	Clinical observation
C	5		0.29			
A	430		25.29			
B	6	17	0.35	Water for injections	Physically stable over 24 h	Clinical observation
C	10		0.59			

Diamorphine (A), Dexamethasone (B) and **Hyoscine Hydrobromide (C)**

Summary: No problems with physical stability encountered. It is usual to give dexamethasone as a subcutaneous bolus injection

Drug	Dose in syringe (mg)	Volume in syringe (ml)	Concentration (mg/ml)	Diluent	Outcome	Data type
A	20		1.33			
B	4	15	0.27	Water for injections	Physically stable over 24 h	Clinical observation
C	1.2		0.08			
A	20		1.33			
B	8	15	0.53	Water for injections	Physically stable over 24 h	Clinical observation
C	0.8		0.05			

Diamorphine (A), Dexamethasone (B) and **Levomepromazine (C)**

Summary: Mixture physically incompatible at the concentrations below; solution becomes turbid. Note that the mixture of dexamethasone and levomepromazine alone has been shown to be incompatible. It is usual to give dexamethasone via a subcutaneous bolus injection. Levomepromazine may be given as a subcutaneous bolus injection at doses below 50 mg (= 2 ml)

Drug	Dose in syringe (mg)	Volume in syringe (ml)	Concentration (mg/ml)	Diluent	Outcome	Data type
A	10		0.50			
B	8	20	0.40	Water for injections	Incompatible	Clinical observation
C	12.5		0.63			
A	120		7.06			
B	10	17	0.59	Water for injections	Incompatible	Clinical observation
C	50		2.94			

Diamorphine (A), Dexamethasone (B) and **Metoclopramide (C)**

Summary: No problems with physical stability encountered, although precipitation/turbidity may occur with higher concentrations of dexamethasone. It is usual to give dexamethasone via a subcutaneous bolus injection

Drug	Dose in syringe (mg)	Volume in syringe (ml)	Concentration (mg/ml)	Diluent	Outcome	Data type
A	30		1.76			
B	12	17	0.71	Water for injections	Physically stable over 24 h	Clinical observation
C	60		3.53			
A	60		3.53			
B	10	17	0.59	Water for injections	Physically stable over 24 h	Clinical observation
C	40		2.35			
A	150		8.82			
B	4	17	0.24	Water for injections	Physically stable over 24 h	Clinical observation
C	30		1.76			
A	100		5.88			
B	4	17	0.24	Water for injections	Physically stable over 24 h	Clinical observation
C	50		2.94			

Diamorphine (A), Dexamethasone (B) and **Midazolam (C)**

Summary: No problems with physical stability encountered, although precipitation or turbidity may occur as concentrations of dexamethasone increase. It is usual to give dexamethasone via a subcutaneous bolus injection

Drug	Dose in syringe (mg)	Volume in syringe (ml)	Concentration (mg/ml)	Diluent	Outcome	Data type
A	50		2.94			
B	4	17	0.24	Water for injections	Physically stable over 24 h	Clinical observation
C	20		1.18			

Diamorphine (A), Dexamethasone (B) and **Ondansetron (C)**

Summary: No problems with physical stability encountered. It is usual to give dexamethasone via a subcutaneous bolus injection

Drug	Dose in syringe (mg)	Volume in syringe (ml)	Concentration (mg/ml)	Diluent	Outcome	Data type
A	600		35.29			
B	1	17	0.06	Water for injections	Physically stable over 24 h	Clinical observation
C	24		1.41			

Diamorphine (A), Glycopyrronium (B) and **Levomepromazine (C)**

Summary: No problems with physical stability encountered. To reduce irritation at the site of infusion, levomepromazine may be given as a subcutaneous bolus injection at doses below 50 mg (= 2 ml)

Drug	Dose in syringe (mg)	Volume in syringe (ml)	Concentration (mg/ml)	Diluent	Outcome	Data type
A	30		1.76			
B	1.6	17	0.05	Water for injections	Physically stable over 24 h	Clinical observation
C	100		0.74			
A			4.12			
B		17	0.09	Water for injections	Physically stable over 24 h	Clinical observation
C			5.88			

Diamorphine (A), Glycopyrronium (B) and **Midazolam (C)**

Summary: No problems with physical stability encountered

Drug	Dose in syringe (mg)	Volume in syringe (ml)	Concentration (mg/ml)	Diluent	Outcome	Data type
A	120		6.67			
B	1.6	17	0.08	Water for injections	Physically stable over 24 h	Clinical observation
C	30		1.33			
A	420		24.71			
B	0.8	17	0.05	Water for injections	Physically stable over 24 h	Clinical observation
C	40		2.35			

Diamorphine (A), Haloperidol (B) and **Hyoscine Butylbromide (C)**

Summary: No problems with physical stability encountered

Drug	Dose in syringe (mg)	Volume in syringe (ml)	Concentration (mg/ml)	Diluent	Outcome	Data type
A	30		1.76			
B	10	17	0.59	Water for injections	Physically stable over 24 h	Clinical observation
C	120		7.06			
A	60		3.53			
B	10	17	0.59	Water for injections	Physically stable over 24 h	Clinical observation
C	80		4.71			
A	180		10.59			
B	5	17	0.29	Water for injections	Physically stable over 24 h	Clinical observation
C	80		4.71			

Diamorphine (A), Haloperidol (B) and **Levomepromazine (C)**

Summary: No problems with physical stability encountered. To reduce irritation at the site of infusion, levomepromazine may be given as a subcutaneous bolus injection at doses below 50 mg (= 2 ml)

Drug	Dose in syringe (mg)	Volume in syringe (ml)	Concentration (mg/ml)	Diluent	Outcome	Data type
A	720		42.35			
B	10	17	0.59	Water for injections	Physically stable over 24 h	Clinical observation
C	200		11.76			

Diamorphine (A), Haloperidol (B) and **Metoclopramide (C)**

Summary: No problems with physical stability encountered. Note, however, that there is usually no need to use this combination

Drug	Dose in syringe (mg)	Volume in syringe (ml)	Concentration (mg/ml)	Diluent	Outcome	Data type
A	40		2.35			
B	5	17	0.29	Water for injections	Physically stable over 24 h	Clinical observation
C	30		1.76			
A	80		4.71			
B	10	17	0.59	Water for injections	Physically stable over 24 h	Clinical observation
C	60		3.53			
A	130		7.65			
B	5	17	0.29	Water for injections	Physically stable over 24 h	Clinical observation
C	60		3.53			

Diamorphine (A), Haloperidol (B) and **Midazolam (C)**

Summary: No problems with physical stability encountered

Drug	Dose in syringe (mg)	Volume in syringe (ml)	Concentration (mg/ml)	Diluent	Outcome	Data type
A	20		1.18	Water for injections	Physically stable over 24 h	Clinical observation
B	5	17	0.29			
C	30		1.76			
A	40		2.35	Water for injections	Physically stable over 24 h	Clinical observation
B	2.5	17	0.15			
C	20		1.18			
A	120		7.06	Water for injections	Physically stable over 24 h	Clinical observation
B	5	17	0.29			
C	30		1.76			
A	450		26.47	Water for injections	Physically stable over 24 h	Clinical observation
B	5	17	0.29			
C	20		1.18			
A	630		37.06	Water for injections	Physically stable over 24 h	Clinical observation
B	10	17	0.59			
C	30		1.76			
A	840		49.41	Water for injections	Physically stable over 24 h	Clinical observation
B	10	17	0.59			
C	40		2.35			

Diamorphine (A), Hyoscine Butylbromide (B) and **Levomepromazine (C)**

Summary: No problems with physical stability encountered. To reduce irritation at the site of infusion, levomepromazine may be given as a subcutaneous bolus injection at doses below 50 mg (= 2 ml)

Drug	Dose in syringe (mg)	Volume in syringe (ml)	Concentration (mg/ml)	Diluent	Outcome	Data type
A	40		2.35			
B	120	17	7.06	Water for injections	Physically stable over 24 h	Clinical observation
C	6.25		0.37			
A	100		5.88			
B	80	17	4.71	Water for injections	Physically stable over 24 h	Clinical observation
C	25		1.47			
A	120		7.06			
B	120	17	7.06	Water for injections	Physically stable over 24 h	Clinical observation
C	50		2.94			
A	350		20.59			
B	80	17	4.71	Water for injections	Physically stable over 24 h	Clinical observation
C	50		2.94			
A	1400		82.35			
B	120	17	7.06	Water for injections	Physically stable over 24 h	Clinical observation
C	37.50		2.21			
A	1900		111.6			
B	120	17	7.06	Water for injections	Physically stable over 24 h	Clinical observation
C	50		2.94			

Diamorphine (A), Hyoscine Hydrobromide (B) and **Levomepromazine (C)**

Summary: No problems with physical stability encountered. To reduce irritation at the site of infusion, levomepromazine may be given as a subcutaneous bolus injection at doses below 50 mg (= 2 ml)

Drug	Dose in syringe (mg)	Volume in syringe (ml)	Concentration (mg/ml)	Diluent	Outcome	Data type
A	80		4.71			
B	1.8	17	0.11	Water for injections	Physically stable over 24 h	Clinical observation
C	75		4.41			
A	450		26.47			
B	2.4	17	0.14	Water for injections	Physically stable over 24 h	Clinical observation
C	100		5.88			

Diamorphine (A), Hyoscine Hydrobromide (B) and **Midazolam (C)**

Summary: No problems with physical stability encountered

Drug	Dose in syringe (mg)	Volume in syringe (ml)	Concentration (mg/ml)	Diluent	Outcome	Data type
A	50		2.94	Water for injections	Physically stable over 24 h	Clinical observation
B	2.4	17	0.14			
C	20		1.18			
A	70		4.12	Water for injections	Physically stable over 24 h	Clinical observation
B	1.2	17	0.07			
C	30		1.76			
A	80		4.71	Water for injections	Physically stable over 24 h	Clinical observation
B	1.6	17	0.09			
C	20		1.18			
A	160		9.41	Water for injections	Physically stable over 24 h	Clinical observation
B	1.2	17	0.07			
C	30		1.76			
A	200		11.76	Water for injections	Physically stable over 24 h	Clinical observation
B	1.2	17	0.07			
C	30		1.76			
A	420		24.71	Water for injections	Physically stable over 24 h	Clinical observation
B	1.6	17	0.09			
C	40		2.35			
A	720		42.35	Water for injections	Physically stable over 24 h	Clinical observation
B	1.6	17	0.09			
C	40		2.35			

Diamorphine (A), Levomepromazine (B) and **Metoclopramide (C)**

Summary: No problems with physical stability encountered. To reduce irritation at the site of infusion, levomepromazine may be given as a subcutaneous bolus injection at doses below 50 mg (= 2 ml). Note that levomepromazine can antagonize the prokinetic effect of metoclopramide

Drug	Dose in syringe (mg)	Volume in syringe (ml)	Concentration (mg/ml)	Diluent	Outcome	Data type
A	70		4.12			
B	12.5	17	0.74	Water for injections	Physically stable over 24 h	Clinical observation
C	40		2.35			
A	250		14.71			
B	50	17	2.94	Water for injections	Physically stable over 24 h	Clinical observation
C	60		3.53			

Diamorphine (A), Levomepromazine (B) and **Midazolam (C)**

Summary: No problems with physical stability encountered. To reduce irritation at the site of infusion, levomepromazine may be given as a subcutaneous bolus injection at doses below 50 mg (= 2 ml)

Drug	Dose in syringe (mg)	Volume in syringe (ml)	Concentration (mg/ml)	Diluent	Outcome	Data type
A	60		3.53			
B	125	17	7.35	Water for injections	Physically stable over 24 h	Clinical observation
C	25		1.47			
A	1450		85.29			
B	12.5	17	0.74	Water for injections	Physically stable over 24 h	Clinical observation
C	30		1.76			
A	1600		94.12			
B	50	17	2.94	Water for injections	Physically stable over 24 h	Clinical observation
C	30		1.76			

Diamorphine (A), Levomepromazine (B) and Octreotide (C)

Summary: No problems with physical stability encountered. To reduce irritation at the site of infusion, levomepromazine may be given as a subcutaneous bolus injection at doses below 50 mg (= 2 ml)

Drug	Dose in syringe (mg)	Volume in syringe (ml)	Concentration (mg/ml)	Diluent	Outcome	Data type
A	50		2.94			
B	37.5	17	2.21	Water for injections	Physically stable over 24 h	Clinical observation
C	0.60		0.04			
A	80		4.71			
B	50	17	2.94	Water for injections	Physically stable over 24 h	Clinical observation
C	0.60		0.04			
A	170		10.00			
B	75	17	4.41	Water for injections	Physically stable over 24 h	Clinical observation
C	1.00		0.06			

Diamorphine (A), Metoclopramide (B) and Midazolam (C)

Summary: No problems with physical stability encountered

Drug	Dose in syringe (mg)	Volume in syringe (ml)	Concentration (mg/ml)	Diluent	Outcome	Data type
A	50		2.94			
B	30	17	1.76	Water for injections	Physically stable over 24 h	Clinical observation
C	10		0.59			
A	180		10.59			
B	20	17	1.18	Water for injections	Physically stable over 24 h	Clinical observation
C	40		2.35			
A	250		14.71			
B	40	17	2.35	Water for injections	Physically stable over 24 h	Clinical observation
C	30		1.76			
A	420		24.71			
B	60	17	3.53	Water for injections	Physically stable over 24 h	Clinical observation
C	20		1.18			

Diamorphine (A), Midazolam (B) and Octreotide (C)

Summary: No problems with physical stability encountered

Drug	Dose in syringe (mg)	Volume in syringe (ml)	Concentration (mg/ml)	Diluent	Outcome	Data type
A	140		8.24			
B	40	17	2.35	Water for injections	Physically stable over 24 h	Clinical observation
C	0.6		0.04			

Dihydrocodeine (A), Glycopyrronium (B) and Midazolam (C)

Summary: No problems with physical stability encountered

Drug	Dose in syringe (mg)	Volume in syringe (ml)	Concentration (mg/ml)	Diluent	Outcome	Data type
A	50		5.00			
B	0.8	10	0.08	Water for injections	Physically stable over 24 h	Clinical observation
C	20		2.00			

Hydromorphone (A), Haloperidol (B) and Hyoscine Hydrobromide (C)

Summary: No problems with physical stability encountered

Drug	Dose in syringe (mg)	Volume in syringe (ml)	Concentration (mg/ml)	Diluent	Outcome	Data type
A	100		14.29			
B	10	7	1.43	Dextrose 5%	Physically stable over 24 h	Laboratory
C	1.2		0.17			

Hydromorphone (A), Hyoscine Hydrobromide (B) and Octreotide (C)

Summary: No problems with physical stability encountered

Drug	Dose in syringe (mg)	Volume in syringe (ml)	Concentration (mg/ml)	Diluent	Outcome	Data type
A	100		18.87			
B	1.2	5.3	0.23	Dextrose 5%	Physically stable over 24 h	Laboratory
C	0.3		0.06			

Hydromorphone (A), Metoclopramide (B) and **Ondansetron (C)**

Summary: No problems with physical stability encountered

Drug	Dose in syringe (mg)	Volume in syringe (ml)	Concentration (mg/ml)	Diluent	Outcome	Data type
A	200		11.11			
B	30	18	1.67	Dextrose 5%	Physically stable over 24 h	Laboratory
C	16		0.89			

Methadone (A), Glycopyrronium (B) and **Midazolam (C)**

Summary: No problems with physical stability encountered

Drug	Dose in syringe (mg)	Volume in syringe (ml)	Concentration (mg/ml)	Diluent	Outcome	Data type
A	40		2.00			
B	1.2	20	0.06	Sodium chloride 0.9%	Physically stable over 24 h	Clinical observation
C	40		2.00			
A	50		2.50			
B	0.8	20	0.04	Sodium chloride 0.9%	Physically stable over 24 h	Clinical observation
C	20		1.00			

Morphine Sulphate (A), Haloperidol (B) and **Hyoscine Hydrobromide (C)**

Summary: No problems with physical stability encountered

Drug	Dose in syringe (mg)	Volume in syringe (ml)	Concentration (mg/ml)	Diluent	Outcome	Data type
A	400		30.77			
B	10	13	0.77	Dextrose 5%	Physically stable over 24 h	Laboratory
C	1.2		0.09			

Morphine Sulphate (A), Hyoscine Hydrobromide (B) and **Octreotide (C)**

Summary: No problems with physical stability encountered

Drug	Dose in syringe (mg)	Volume in syringe (ml)	Concentration (mg/ml)	Diluent	Outcome	Data type
A	400		35.40			
B	1.2	11.3	0.11	Dextrose 5%	Physically stable over 24 h	Laboratory
C	0.3		0.03			

Morphine Sulphate (A), Metoclopramide (B) and **Ondansetron (C)**

Summary: No problems with physical stability encountered

Drug	Dose in syringe (mg)	Volume in syringe (ml)	Concentration (mg/ml)	Diluent	Outcome	Data type
A	400		18.18			
B	30	22	1.36	Dextrose 5%	Physically stable over 24 h	Laboratory
C	16		0.73			

Clonazepam (A), Haloperidol (B) and **Metoclopramide (C)**

Summary: No problems with physical stability encountered

Drug	Dose in syringe (mg)	Volume in syringe (ml)	Concentration (mg/ml)	Diluent	Outcome	Data type
A	4		0.24			
B	10	17	0.59	Water for injections	Physically stable over 24 h	Clinical observation
C	30		1.76			

Cyclizine (A), Dexamethasone (B) and **Hyoscine Butylbromide (C)**

Summary: Cyclizine may crystallize with hyoscine butylbromide. If an anticholinergic drug is required, hyoscine hydrobromide is an acceptable alternative in this case. It is usual to give dexamethasone via subcutaneous bolus injection

Drug	Dose in syringe (mg)	Volume in syringe (ml)	Concentration (mg/ml)	Diluent	Outcome	Data type
A	150		8.82			
B	12	17	0.71	Water for injections	Physically stable over 24 h	Clinical observation
C	40		2.35			

Cyclizine (A), Haloperidol (B) and **Midazolam (C)**

Summary: No problems with physical stability encountered

Drug	Dose in syringe (mg)	Volume in syringe (ml)	Concentration (mg/ml)	Diluent	Outcome	Data type
A	150		8.82			
B	5	17	0.29	Water for injections	Physically stable over 24 h	Clinical observation
C	30		1.76			

Glycopyrronium (A), Levomepromazine (B) and **Octreotide (C)**

Summary: No problems with physical stability encountered. To reduce irritation at the site of infusion, levomepromazine may be given as a subcutaneous bolus injection at doses below 50 mg (= 2 ml)

Drug	Dose in syringe (mg)	Volume in syringe (ml)	Concentration (mg/ml)	Diluent	Outcome	Data type
A	1.6		0.09			
B	25	17	1.47	Water for injections	Physically stable over 24 h	Clinical observation
C	0.6		0.04			

Haloperidol (A), Hyoscine Butylbromide (B) and **Midazolam (C)**

Summary: No problems with physical stability encountered.

Drug	Dose in syringe (mg)	Volume in syringe (ml)	Concentration (mg/ml)	Diluent	Outcome	Data type
A	5		0.30	Water for injections	Physically stable over 24 h	Clinical observation
B	180	16.5	10.91			
C	10		0.61			

Hyoscine Hydrobromide (A), Ketorolac (B) and **Ranitidine (C)**

Summary: No problems with physical stability encountered

Drug	Dose in syringe (mg)	Volume in syringe (ml)	Concentration (mg/ml)	Diluent	Outcome	Data type
A	0.8		0.04	Sodium chloride 0.9%	Physically stable over 24 h	Clinical observation
B	90	20	4.50			
C	150		7.50			

Levomepromazine (A), Hyoscine Hydrobromide (B) and **Midazolam (C)**

Summary: No problems with physical stability encountered. To reduce irritation at the site of infusion, levomepromazine may be given as a subcutaneous bolus injection at doses below 50 mg (= 2 ml)

Drug	Dose in syringe (mg)	Volume in syringe (ml)	Concentration (mg/ml)	Diluent	Outcome	Data type
A	50		2.94	Water for injections	Physically stable over 24 h	Clinical observation
B	2.4	17	0.14			
C	40		2.35			

Drug A	B	C	D	page
Alfentanil	Clonazepam	Dexamethasone	Haloperidol	120
Alfentanil	Clonazepam	Glycopyrronium	Haloperidol	120
Alfentanil	Cyclizine	Glycopyrronium	Midazolam	121
Alfentanil	Cyclizine	Haloperidol	Octreotide	121
Alfentanil	Dexamethasone	Haloperidol	Midazolam	121
Diamorphine	Clonazepam	Cyclizine	Glycopyrronium	122
Diamorphine	Clonazepam	Cyclizine	Haloperidol	122
Diamorphine	Clonazepam	Dexamethasone	Haloperidol	122
Diamorphine	Clonazepam	Dexamethasone	Hyoscine Hydrobromide	123
Diamorphine	Clonazepam	Glycopyrronium	Haloperidol	123
Diamorphine	Clonazepam	Haloperidol	Hyoscine Hydrobromide	124
Diamorphine	Clonazepam	Hyoscine Butylbromide	Midazolam	124
Diamorphine	Clonazepam	Hyoscine Hydrobromide	Levomepromazine	124
Diamorphine	Cyclizine	Dexamethasone	Haloperidol	125
Diamorphine	Cyclizine	Dexamethasone	Hyoscine Hydrobromide	126
Diamorphine	Cyclizine	Dexamethasone	Metoclopramide	127
Diamorphine	Cyclizine	Glycopyrronium	Haloperidol	128
Diamorphine	Cyclizine	Glycopyrronium	Midazolam	128
Diamorphine	Cyclizine	Haloperidol	Hyoscine Butylbromide	129
Diamorphine	Cyclizine	Haloperidol	Hyoscine Hydrobromide	129
Diamorphine	Cyclizine	Haloperidol	Midazolam	130
Diamorphine	Cyclizine	Haloperidol	Octreotide	130
Diamorphine	Cyclizine	Hyoscine Butylbromide	Midazolam	131
Diamorphine	Cyclizine	Hyoscine Hydrobromide	Metoclopramide	131
Diamorphine	Cyclizine	Hyoscine Hydrobromide	Midazolam	132

Compatibility data tables

Four drugs

Drug A	B	C	D	page
Diamorphine	Cyclizine	Midazolam	Ranitidine	133
Diamorphine	Dexamethasone	Haloperidol	Hyoscine Butylbromide	133
Diamorphine	Dexamethasone	Haloperidol	Levomepromazine	134
Diamorphine	Dexamethasone	Haloperidol	Metoclopramide	134
Diamorphine	Dexamethasone	Hyoscine Hydrobromide	Midazolam	135
Diamorphine	Glycopyrronium	Haloperidol	Midazolam	136
Diamorphine	Glycopyrronium	Levomepromazine	Octreotide	136
Diamorphine	Glycopyrronium	Metoclopramide	Midazolam	137
Diamorphine	Haloperidol	Hyoscine Butylbromide	Levomepromazine	137
Diamorphine	Haloperidol	Levomepromazine	Midazolam	137
Diamorphine	Hyoscine Butylbromide	Levomepromazine	Midazolam	138
Diamorphine	Hyoscine Butylbromide	Levomepromazine	Octreotide	138
Diamorphine	Levomepromazine	Midazolam	Octreotide	139
Hydromorphone	Glycopyrronium	Haloperidol	Promethazine	139
Hydromorphone	Glycopyrronium	Haloperidol	Octreotide	139
Hydromorphone	Glycopyrronium	Metoclopramide	Octreotide	140
Hydromorphone	Haloperidol	Hyoscine Hydrobromide	Promethazine	140
Hydromorphone	Hyoscine Hydrobromide	Metoclopramide	Octreotide	140
Morphine Sulphate	Glycopyrronium	Haloperidol	Promethazine	141
Morphine Sulphate	Glycopyrronium	Haloperidol	Octreotide	141
Morphine Sulphate	Glycopyrronium	Metoclopramide	Octreotide	141
Morphine Sulphate	Haloperidol	Hyoscine Hydrobromide	Promethazine	142
Morphine Sulphate	Hyoscine Hydrobromide	Metoclopramide	Octreotide	142
Cyclizine	Haloperidol	Glycopyrronium	Octreotide	143

Alfentanil (A), Clonazepam (B), Dexamethasone (C) and **Haloperidol (D)**

Summary: No problems with physical stability encountered, although precipitation/turbidity may occur as doses increase (pH effect). Note that a similar reaction occurs with dexamethasone and haloperidol. Dexamethasone is usually given as a subcutaneous bolus injection

Drug	Dose in syringe (mg)	Volume in syringe (ml)	Concentration (mg/ml)	Diluent	Outcome	Data type
A	2		0.12			
B	4	17	0.24	Water for	Physically stable	Clinical
C	16		0.94	injections	over 24 h	observation
D	3		0.18			

Alfentanil (A), Clonazepam (B), Glycopyrronium (C) and **Haloperidol (D)**

Summary: No problems with physical stability encountered

Drug	Dose in syringe (mg)	Volume in syringe (ml)	Concentration (mg/ml)	Diluent	Outcome	Data type
A	3		0.20			
B	2	15	0.13	Water for	Physically stable	Clinical
C	0.8		0.05	injections	over 24 h	observation
D	5		0.33			

Alfentanil (A), Cyclizine (B), Glycopyrronium (C) and **Midazolam (D)**

Summary: No problems with physical stability encountered. Crystallisation may occur as concentrations increase.

Drug	Dose in syringe (mg)	Volume in syringe (ml)	Concentration (mg/ml)	Diluent	Outcome	Data type
A	4		0.24			
B	150	17	8.82	Water for	Physically stable	Clinical
C	0.8		0.05	injections	over 24 h	observation
D	10		0.59			
A	5		0.38			
B	100	13	7.69	Water for	Physically stable	Clinical
C	0.6		0.05	injections	over 24 h	observation
D	10		0.77			

Alfentanil (A), Cyclizine (B), Haloperidol (C) and **Octreotide (D)**

Summary: No problems with physical stability encountered. Crystallisation may occur as concentrations increase.

Drug	Dose in syringe (mg)	Volume in syringe (ml)	Concentration (mg/ml)	Diluent	Outcome	Data type
A	10		0.63			
B	150	16	9.38	Water for	Physically stable	Clinical
C	10		0.63	injections	over 24 h	observation
D	0.6		0.04			

Alfentanil (A), Dexamethasone (B), Haloperidol (C) and **Midazolam (D)**

Summary: Physically incompatible; immediate turbidity. Note that a similar reaction occurs with dexamethasone and haloperidol. To overcome this problem, dexamethasone should be given via a subcutaneous bolus injection, or separate CSCI

Drug	Dose in syringe (mg)	Volume in syringe (ml)	Concentration (mg/ml)	Diluent	Outcome	Data type
A	4.5		0.26			
B	16	17	0.94	Water for	Incompatible	Clinical
C	3		0.18	injections		observation
D	20		1.18			

Diamorphine (A), Clonazepam (B), Cyclizine (C) and **Glycopyrronium (D)**

Summary: No problems with physical stability encountered. Crystallisation may occur as concentrations increase.

Drug	Dose in syringe (mg)	Volume in syringe (ml)	Concentration (mg/ml)	Diluent	Outcome	Data type
A	100		5.88			
B	4	17	0.24	Water for injections	Physically stable over 24 h	Clinical observation
C	150		8.82			
D	1.2		0.07			

Diamorphine (A), Clonazepam (B), Cyclizine (C) and **Haloperidol (D)**

Summary: No problems with physical stability encountered. Crystallisation may occur as concentrations increase.

Drug	Dose in syringe (mg)	Volume in syringe (ml)	Concentration (mg/ml)	Diluent	Outcome	Data type
A	40		2.35			
B	2	17	0.12	Water for injections	Physically stable over 24 h	Clinical observation
C	150		8.82			
D	5		0.29			

Diamorphine (A), Clonazepam (B), **Dexamethasone (C)** and **Haloperidol (D)**

Summary: No problems with physical stability encountered, although precipitation/turbidity may occur as doses increase. Note that a similar reaction occurs with dexamethasone and haloperidol. To overcome this, dexamethasone should be given via a bolus subcutaneous injection, or separate CSCI. Alternatively, either haloperidol or clonazepam may be given by subcutaneous bolus injection

Drug	Dose in syringe (mg)	Volume in syringe (ml)	Concentration (mg/ml)	Diluent	Outcome	Data type
A	5		0.29			
B	2	17	0.12	Water for injections	Physically stable over 24 h	Clinical observation
C	12		0.71			
D	5		0.29			

Diamorphine (A), Clonazepam (B), Dexamethasone (C) and Hyoscine Hydrobromide (D)

Summary: No problems with physical stability encountered. Problems may occur with higher doses of dexamethasone. This can be overcome by giving the dexamethasone via a subcutaneous bolus injection, or separate CSCI. Alternatively, clonazepam can be given as a subcutaneous bolus injection, although the dose may make this impractical

Drug	Dose in syringe (mg)	Volume in syringe (ml)	Concentration (mg/ml)	Diluent	Outcome	Data type
A	20		1.18			
B	4	17	0.24	Water for injections	Physically stable over 24 h	Clinical observation
C	8		0.47			
D	0.11		0.11			

Diamorphine (A), Clonazepam (B), Glycopyrronium (C) and Haloperidol (D)

Summary: No problems with physical stability encountered

Drug	Dose in syringe (mg)	Volume in syringe (ml)	Concentration (mg/ml)	Diluent	Outcome	Data type
A	130		7.65			
B	4	17	0.24	Water for injections	Physically stable over 24 h	Clinical observation
C	0.4		0.02			
D	5		0.29			
A	120		12.00			
B	2	10	0.20	Water for injections	Physically stable over 24 h	Clinical observation
C	0.8		0.08			
D	5		0.50			

Diamorphine (A), Clonazepam (B), Haloperidol (C) and Hyoscine Hydrobromide (D)

Summary: No problems with physical stability encountered

Drug	Dose in syringe (mg)	Volume in syringe (ml)	Concentration (mg/ml)	Diluent	Outcome	Data type
A	120		8.00			
B	6	15	0.40	Water for	Physically stable	Clinical
C	5		0.33	injections	over 24 h	observation
D	1.2		0.08			

Diamorphine (A), Clonazepam (B), Hyoscine Butylbromide (C) and Midazolam (D)

Summary: No problems with physical stability encountered

Drug	Dose in syringe (mg)	Volume in syringe (ml)	Concentration (mg/ml)	Diluent	Outcome	Data type
A	1800		102.6			
B	3	17.5	0.17	Water for	Physically stable	Clinical
C	120		6.86	injections	over 24 h	observation
D	10		0.57			

Diamorphine (A), Clonazepam (B), Hyoscine Hydrobromide (C) and Levomepromazine (D)

Summary: No problems with physical stability encountered. To reduce irritation at the site of infusion, levomepromazine may be given as a subcutaneous bolus injection at doses below 50 mg (= 2 ml)

Drug	Dose in syringe (mg)	Volume in syringe (ml)	Concentration (mg/ml)	Diluent	Outcome	Data type
A	60		3.53			
B	4	17	0.24	Water for	Physically stable	Clinical
C	1.6		0.09	injections	over 24 h	observation
D	50		2.94			

Diamorphine (A), Cyclizine (B), Dexamethasone (C) and **Haloperidol (D)**

Summary: No problems with physical stability encountered, although precipitation/turbidity may occur as doses increase. Note that a similar reaction occurs with dexamethasone and haloperidol. To overcome this, dexamethasone should be given via a bolus subcutaneous injection, or separate CSCI. Alternatively, haloperidol can be given as bolus subcutaneous injection, depending upon dose

Drug	Dose in syringe (mg)	Volume in syringe (ml)	Concentration (mg/ml)	Diluent	Outcome	Data type
A	40		2.35			
B	150	17	8.82	Water for injections	Physically stable over 24 h	Clinical observation
C	4		0.24			
D	5		0.29			
A	70		4.12			
B	150	17	8.82	Water for injections	Physically stable over 24 h	Clinical observation
C	8		0.47			
D	5		0.29			
A	40		5.00			
B	150	8	18.75	Water for injections	Physically stable over 24 h	Clinical observation
C	1		0.13			
D	5		0.63			
A	90		5.29			
B	150	17	8.82	Water for injections	Physically stable over 24 h	Clinical observation
C	8		0.47			
D	10		0.59			
A	450		26.47			
B	150	17	8.82	Water for injections	Physically stable over 24 h	Clinical observation
C	8		0.47			
D	5		0.29			

Diamorphine (A), Cyclizine (B), Dexamethasone (C) and **Hyoscine Hydrobromide (D)**

Summary: No problems with physical stability encountered, although precipitation/turbidity may occur as doses increase. Note that dexamethasone should usually be given via a bolus subcutaneous injection, or separate CSCI

Drug	Dose in syringe (mg)	Volume in syringe (ml)	Concentration (mg/ml)	Diluent	Outcome	Data type
A	60		3.53			
B	150	17	8.82	Water for injections	Physically stable over 24 h	Clinical observation
C	8		0.47			
D	1.8		0.11			

Diamorphine (A), Cyclizine (B), Dexamethasone (C) and Metoclopramide (D)

Summary: Crystallization may occur as concentrations increase. This is **not** a sensible combination of antiemetics, since the prokinetic action of metoclopramide is inhibited by cyclizine. Higher doses of metoclopramide will be required to overcome this. However, use of this combination is acceptable if metoclopramide is used for its central dopamine antagonist properties. Note that dexamethasone should normally be given via a bolus subcutaneous injection, or separate CSCI

Drug	Dose in syringe (mg)	Volume in syringe (ml)	Concentration (mg/ml)	Diluent	Outcome	Data type
A	50		2.94			
B	50	17	8.82	Water for injections	Physically stable over 24 h	Clinical observation
C	6		0.35			
D	30		1.76			
A	80		4.71			
B	150	17	8.82	Water for injections	Physically stable over 24 h	Clinical observation
C	2		0.12			
D	30		1.76			
A	190		11.88			
B	150	16	9.38	Water for injections	Incompatible	Clinical observation
C	4		0.25			
D	30		1.88			
A	240		14.12			
B	150	17	8.82	Water for injections	Incompatible	Clinical observation
C	4		0.24			
D	30		1.76			

Diamorphine (A), Cyclizine (B), Glycopyrronium (C) and **Haloperidol (D)**

Summary: No problems with physical stability encountered. Crystallisation may occur as concentrations increase.

Drug	Dose in syringe (mg)	Volume in syringe (ml)	Concentration (mg/ml)	Diluent	Outcome	Data type
A	120		6.67			
B	150	18	8.33	Water for injections	Physically stable over 24 h	Clinical observation
C	2.4		0.13			
D	10		0.56			
A	200		11.76			
B	150	17	8.82	Water for injections	Physically stable over 24 h	Clinical observation
C	0.8		0.05			
D	5		0.29			

Diamorphine (A), Cyclizine (B), Glycopyrronium (C) and **Midazolam (D)**

Summary: This combination may crystallise as concentrations increase. This mixture should be diluted maximally to overcome any problems

Drug	Dose in syringe (mg)	Volume in syringe (ml)	Concentration (mg/ml)	Diluent	Outcome	Data type
A	10		0.59			
B	150	17	8.82	Water for injections	Physically stable over 24 h	Clinical observation
C	1.6		0.09			
D	10		0.59			
A	10		0.50			
B	150	20	7.50	Water for injections	Incompatible	Clinical observation
C	2.4		0.12			
D	15		0.75			
A	20		2.22			
B	150	9	16.67	Water for injections	Incompatible	Clinical observation
C	0.6		0.07			
D	10		1.11			
A	100		6.67			
B	150	15	10.00	Water for injections	Physically stable over 24 h	Clinical observation
C	1.2		0.08			
D	20		1.33			

Diamorphine (A), Cyclizine (B), Haloperidol (C) and **Hyoscine Butylbromide (D)**

Summary: This mixture is likely to be physically incompatible. Combination may crystallize as concentrations increase

Drug	Dose in syringe (mg)	Volume in syringe (ml)	Concentration (mg/ml)	Diluent	Outcome	Data type
A	60		3.53			
B	150	17	8.82	Water for injections	Incompatible	Clinical observation
C	10		0.59			
D	80		4.71			
A	120		7.06			
B	75	17	4.41	Water for injections	Physically stable over 24 h	Clinical observation
C	2.5		0.15			
D	40		2.35			
A	320		18.82			
B	150	17	8.82	Water for injections	Incompatible	Clinical observation
C	10		0.59			
D	120		7.06			

Diamorphine (A), Cyclizine (B), Haloperidol (C) and **Hyoscine Hydrobromide (D)**

Summary: No problems with physical stability encountered. Combination may crystallise as concentrations increase

Drug	Dose in syringe (mg)	Volume in syringe (ml)	Concentration (mg/ml)	Diluent	Outcome	Data type
A	230		13.53			
B	150	17	8.82	Water for injections	Physically stable over 24 h	Clinical observation
C	10		0.59			
D	1.6		0.09			

Diamorphine (A), Cyclizine (B), Haloperidol (C) and **Midazolam (D)**

Summary: No problems with physical stability encountered. Combination may crystallise as concentrations increase

Drug	Dose in syringe (mg)	Volume in syringe (ml)	Concentration (mg/ml)	Diluent	Outcome	Data type
A	50		3.57			
B	150	17	10.71	Water for	Physically stable	Clinical
C	5		0.36	injections	over 24 h	observation
D	20		1.43			
A	120		7.06			
B	150	17	10.71	Water for	Physically stable	Clinical
C	5		0.36	injections	over 24 h	observation
D	10		0.59			
A	240		14.12			
B	150	17	8.82	Water for	Physically stable	Clinical
C	10		0.59	injections	over 24 h	observation
D	30		1.76			

Diamorphine (A), Cyclizine (B), Haloperidol (C) and **Octreotide (D)**

Summary: No problems with physical stability encountered. Combination may crystallise as concentrations increase

Drug	Dose in syringe (mg)	Volume in syringe (ml)	Concentration (mg/ml)	Diluent	Outcome	Data type
A	30		1.76			
B	150	17	8.82	Water for	Physically stable	Clinical
C	10		0.59	injections	over 24 h	observation
D	0.6		0.04			
A	130		1.76			
B	150	20	7.50	Water for	Physically stable	Clinical
C	10		0.50	injections	over 24 h	observation
D	0.6		0.03			

Diamorphine (A), Cyclizine (B), Hyoscine Butylbromide (C) and Midazolam (D)

Summary: This mixture is likely to be physically incompatible. Combination may crystallize as concentrations increase

Drug	Dose in syringe (mg)	Volume in syringe (ml)	Concentration (mg/ml)	Diluent	Outcome	Data type
A	30		1.50			
B	150	20	7.50	Water for injections	Incompatible	Clinical observation
C	100		5.00			
D	20		1.00			
A	150		8.82			
B	150	17	8.82	Water for injections	Incompatible	Clinical observation
C	80		4.71			
D	20		1.18			

Diamorphine (A), Cyclizine (B), Hyoscine Hydrobromide (C) and Metoclopramide (D)

Summary: Crystallization is possible at higher concentrations. This mixture should be diluted maximally to overcome any problems

Drug	Dose in syringe (mg)	Volume in syringe (ml)	Concentration (mg/ml)	Diluent	Outcome	Data type
A	170		10.00			
B	150	17	8.82	Water for injections	Physically stable over 24 h	Clinical observation
C	1.2		0.07			
D	30		1.76			

Diamorphine (A), Cyclizine (B), Hyoscine Hydrobromide (C) and Midazolam (D)

Summary: No problems with physical stability encountered. Combination may crystallise as concentrations increase

Drug	Dose in syringe (mg)	Volume in syringe (ml)	Concentration (mg/ml)	Diluent	Outcome	Data type
A	30		1.76			
B	150	17	8.82	Water for injections	Physically stable over 24 h	Clinical observation
C	1.2		0.07			
D	30		1.76			
A	40		2.35			
B	150	17	8.82	Water for injections	Physically stable over 24 h	Clinical observation
C	2.4		0.14			
D	40		2.35			
A	45		2.65			
B	150	17	8.82	Water for injections	Physically stable over 24 h	Clinical observation
C	1.6		0.09			
D	30		1.76			
A	120		7.06			
B	150	17	8.82	Water for injections	Physically stable over 24 h	Clinical observation
C	1.6		0.09			
D	30		1.76			
A	160		8.00			
B	150	20	7.50	Water for injections	Physically stable over 24 h	Clinical observation
C	1.8		0.09			
D	50		2.50			

Diamorphine (A), Cyclizine (B), Midazolam (C) and **Ranitidine (D)**

Summary: No problems with physical stability encountered. Combination may crystallise as concentrations increase

Drug	Dose in syringe (mg)	Volume in syringe (ml)	Concentration (mg/ml)	Diluent	Outcome	Data type
A	10		0.50			
B	150	20	7.50	Water for injections	Physically stable over 24 h	Clinical observation
C	10		0.50			
D	150		7.50			

Diamorphine (A), Dexamethasone (B), Haloperidol (C) and **Hyoscine Butylbromide (D)**

Summary: No problems with physical stability encountered, although precipitation/turbidity may occur as concentrations increase. Note that a similar reaction occurs with dexamethasone and haloperidol. To overcome this, dexamethasone should be given via a bolus subcutaneous injection, or separate CSCI. At low doses, haloperidol may also be given via bolus subcutaneous injection if necessary

Drug	Dose in syringe (mg)	Volume in syringe (ml)	Concentration (mg/ml)	Diluent	Outcome	Data type
A	70		4.12			
B	8	17	0.47	Water for injections	Physically stable over 24 h	Clinical observation
C	5		0.29			
D	80		4.71			

Diamorphine (A), Dexamethasone (B), Haloperidol (C) and Levomepromazine (D)

Summary: Combination likely to be physically incompatible. Note that similar reactions are possible with dexamethasone and haloperidol or levomepromazine. This may be overcome by discontinuing haloperidol and by giving the dexamethasone via a subcutaneous bolus injection, or separate CSCI. Haloperidol and levomepromazine should not usually be given together. Levomepromazine and haloperidol may also be given as a subcutaneous injection at low doses

Drug	Dose in syringe (mg)	Volume in syringe (ml)	Concentration (mg/ml)	Diluent	Outcome	Data type
A	90		5.29			
B	6	17	0.35	Water for injections	**Incompatible**	Clinical observation
C	10		0.59			
D	25		1.47			

Diamorphine (A), Dexamethasone (B), Haloperidol (C) and Metoclopramide (D)

Summary: No problems with physical stability encountered, although precipitation/turbidity may occur as concentrations increase. Note that a similar reaction occurs with dexamethasone and haloperidol. To overcome this, dexamethasone should be given via a bolus subcutaneous injection, or separate CSCI. Metoclopramide and haloperidol should not be used together as antiemetics

Drug	Dose in syringe (mg)	Volume in syringe (ml)	Concentration (mg/ml)	Diluent	Outcome	Data type
A	120		7.06			
B	8	17	0.47	Water for injections	Physically stable over 24 h	Clinical observation
C	10		0.59			
D	30		1.76			
A	260		15.29			
B	6	17	0.35	Water for injections	Physically stable over 24 h	Clinical observation
C	5		0.29			
D	30		1.76			

Diamorphine (A), Dexamethasone (B), Hyoscine Hydrobromide (C) and Midazolam (D)

Summary: No problems with physical stability encountered, although precipitation/turbidity may occur as concentrations increase. To overcome this, dexamethasone should be given via a bolus subcutaneous injection, or separate CSCI

Drug	Dose in syringe (mg)	Volume in syringe (ml)	Concentration (mg/ml)	Diluent	Outcome	Data type
A	30		1.76			
B	4	17	0.24	Water for injections	Physically stable over 24 h	Clinical observation
C	1.8		0.11			
D	15		0.88			
A	70		4.12			
B	8	17	0.47	Water for injections	Physically stable over 24 h	Clinical observation
C	1.2		0.07			
D	30		1.76			
A	120		7.06			
B	8	17	0.47	Water for injections	Physically stable over 24 h	Clinical observation
C	1.6		0.09			
D	20		1.18			

Diamorphine (A), Glycopyrronium (B), Haloperidol (C) and Midazolam (D)

Summary: No problems with physical stability encountered

Drug	Dose in syringe (mg)	Volume in syringe (ml)	Concentration (mg/ml)	Diluent	Outcome	Data type
A	45		2.65			
B	1.2	17	0.07	Water for	Physically stable	Clinical
C	10		0.59	injections	over 24 h	observation
D	20		1.18			
A	90		5.29			
B	0.8	17	0.05	Water for	Physically stable	Clinical
C	5		0.29	injections	over 24 h	observation
D	30		1.76			
A	130		7.65			
B	1.6	17	0.09	Water for	Physically stable	Clinical
C	10		0.59	injections	over 24 h	observation
D	20		1.18			

Diamorphine (A), Glycopyrronium (B), Levomepromazine (C) and Octreotide (D)

Summary: No problems with physical stability encountered. To prevent any irritation at the site of infusion, levomepromazine may be given as a subcutaneous injection at doses below 50 mg (= 2 ml)

Drug	Dose in syringe (mg)	Volume in syringe (ml)	Concentration (mg/ml)	Diluent	Outcome	Data type
A	20		1.18			
B	1.8	17	0.11	Water for	Physically stable	Clinical
C	50		2.94	injections	over 24 h	observation
D	0.6		0.04			
A	40		2.00			
B	1.6	20	0.08	Water for	Physically stable	Clinical
C	12.5		0.63	injections	over 24 h	observation
D	0.6		0.03			
A	100		5.88			
B	2.4	17	0.14	Water for	Physically stable	Clinical
C	50		2.94	injections	over 24 h	observation
D	0.6		0.04			

Diamorphine (A), Glycopyrronium (B), Metoclopramide (C) and Midazolam (D)

Summary: No problems with physical stability encountered

Drug	Dose in syringe (mg)	Volume in syringe (ml)	Concentration (mg/ml)	Diluent	Outcome	Data type
A	40		2.35			
B	1.2	17	0.07	Water for injections	Physically stable over 24 h	Clinical observation
C	40		2.35			
D	30		1.76			

Diamorphine (A), Haloperidol (B), Hyoscine Butylbromide (C) and Levomepromazine (D)

Summary: No problems with physical stability encountered. Note that it is not usually necessary to give both haloperidol and levomepromazine together. To prevent site irritation, levomepromazine may be given as a subcutaneous injection at doses below 50 mg (= 2 ml)

Drug	Dose in syringe (mg)	Volume in syringe (ml)	Concentration (mg/ml)	Diluent	Outcome	Data type
A	40		2.35			
B	10	17	0.59	Water for injections	Physically stable over 24 h	Clinical observation
C	80		4.71			
D	25		1.47			

Diamorphine (A), Haloperidol (B), Levomepromazine (C) and Midazolam (D)

Summary: No problems with physical stability encountered. Note that it is normally not necessary to use haloperidol and levomepromazine together. Levomepromazine may also be given as a subcutaneous injection at doses below 50 mg (= 2 ml)

Drug	Dose in syringe (mg)	Volume in syringe (ml)	Concentration (mg/ml)	Diluent	Outcome	Data type
A	320		18.82			
B	10	17	0.59	Water for injections	Physically stable over 24 h	Clinical observation
C	150		8.82			
D	20		1.18			

Diamorphine (A), Hyoscine Butylbromide (B), Levomepromazine (C) and Midazolam (D)

Summary: No problems with physical stability encountered. To prevent irritation at the site of infusion, levomepromazine may be given as a subcutaneous injection at doses below 50 mg (= 2 ml)

Drug	Dose in syringe (mg)	Volume in syringe (ml)	Concentration (mg/ml)	Diluent	Outcome	Data type
A	120		7.06			
B	80	17	4.71	Water for	Physically stable	Clinical
C	25		1.47	injections	over 24 h	observation
D	20		1.18			
A	730		42.94			
B	90	17	5.29	Water for	Physically stable	Clinical
C	50		2.94	injections	over 24 h	observation
D	10		0.59			

Diamorphine (A), Hyoscine Butylbromide (B), Levomepromazine (C) and Octreotide (D)

Summary: No problems with physical stability encountered. To prevent irritation at the site of infusion, levomepromazine may be given as a subcutaneous injection at doses below 50 mg (= 2 ml)

Drug	Dose in syringe (mg)	Volume in syringe (ml)	Concentration (mg/ml)	Diluent	Outcome	Data type
A	40		2.35			
B	90	17	5.29	Water for	Physically stable	Clinical
C	25		1.47	injections	over 24 h	observation
D	0.6		0.04			
A	50		2.94			
B	60	17	3.53	Water for	Physically stable	Clinical
C	50		2.94	injections	over 24 h	observation
D	0.6		0.04			

Diamorphine (A), Levomepromazine (B), Midazolam (C) and Octreotide (D)

Summary: No problems with physical stability encountered

Drug	Dose in syringe (mg)	Volume in syringe (ml)	Concentration (mg/ml)	Diluent	Outcome	Data type
A	40		2.35			
B	12.5	17	0.74	Water for injections	Physically stable over 24 h	Clinical observation
C	20		1.18			
D	0.5		0.03			

Hydromorphone (A), Glycopyrronium (B), Haloperidol (C) and Promethazine (D)

Summary: No problems with physical stability encountered, although haloperidol and promethazine should not normally be given together

Drug	Dose in syringe (mg)	Volume in syringe (ml)	Concentration (mg/ml)	Diluent	Outcome	Data type
A	250		12.5			
B	2.4	20	0.12	Dextrose 5%	Physically stable over 24 h	Laboratory
C	5		0.25			
D	100		5.00			

Hydromorphone (A), Glycopyrronium (B), Haloperidol (C) and Octreotide (D)

Summary: No problems with physical stability encountered

Drug	Dose in syringe (mg)	Volume in syringe (ml)	Concentration (mg/ml)	Diluent	Outcome	Data type
A	100		9.71			
B	1.2	10.3	0.12	Dextrose 5%	Physically stable over 24 h	Laboratory
C	10		0.97			
D	0.3		0.03			

Hydromorphone (A), Glycopyrronium (B), Metoclopramide (C) and Octreotide (D)

Summary: No problems with physical stability encountered

Drug	Dose in syringe (mg)	Volume in syringe (ml)	Concentration (mg/ml)	Diluent	Outcome	Data type
A	100		6.99			
B	1.2	14.3	0.08	Dextrose 5%	Physically stable over 24 h	Laboratory
C	30		2.10			
D	0.3		0.02			

Hydromorphone (A), Haloperidol (B), Hyoscine Hydrobromide (C) and Promethazine (D)

Summary: Physically incompatible at these concentrations

Drug	Dose in syringe (mg)	Volume in syringe (ml)	Concentration (mg/ml)	Diluent	Outcome	Data type
A	100		12.5			
B	10	8	1.25	Dextrose 5%	**Incompatible**	Laboratory
C	1.2		0.15			
D	50		6.25			

Hydromorphone (A), Hyoscine Hydrobromide (B), Metoclopramide (C) and Octreotide (D)

Summary: No problems with physical stability encountered

Drug	Dose in syringe (mg)	Volume in syringe (ml)	Concentration (mg/ml)	Diluent	Outcome	Data type
A	100		8.85			
B	1.2	11.3	0.11	Dextrose 5%	Physically stable over 24 h	Laboratory
C	30		2.65			
D	0.3		0.03			

Morphine Sulphate (A), Glycopyrronium (B), Haloperidol (C) and Promethazine (D)

Summary: No problems with physical stability encountered, although haloperidol and promethazine should not normally be given together

Drug	Dose in syringe (mg)	Volume in syringe (ml)	Concentration (mg/ml)	Diluent	Outcome	Data type
A	400		22.22			
B	2.4	18	0.13	Dextrose 5%	Physically stable over 24 h	Laboratory
C	5		0.28			
D	100		5.56			

Morphine Sulphate (A), Glycopyrronium (B), Haloperidol (C) and Octreotide (D)

Summary: No problems with physical stability encountered

Drug	Dose in syringe (mg)	Volume in syringe (ml)	Concentration (mg/ml)	Diluent	Outcome	Data type
A	400		24.54			
B	1.2	16.3	0.07	Dextrose 5%	Physically stable over 24 h	Laboratory
C	10		0.61			
D	0.3		0.02			

Morphine Sulphate (A), Glycopyrronium (B), Metoclopramide (C) and Octreotide (D)

Summary: No problems with physical stability encountered

Drug	Dose in syringe (mg)	Volume in syringe (ml)	Concentration (mg/ml)	Diluent	Outcome	Data type
A	400		19.70			
B	1.2	20.3	0.06	Dextrose 5%	Physically stable over 24 h	Laboratory
C	30		1.48			
D	0.3		0.01			

Morphine Sulphate (A), Haloperidol (B), Hyoscine Hydrobromide (C) and Promethazine (D)

Summary: Physically incompatible at these concentrations

Drug	Dose in syringe (mg)	Volume in syringe (ml)	Concentration (mg/ml)	Diluent	Outcome	Data type
A	400		28.57			
B	10	14	0.71	Dextrose 5%	Incompatible	Laboratory
C	1.2		0.09			
D	50		3.57			

Morphine Sulphate (A), Hyoscine Hydrobromide (B), Metoclopramide (C) and Octreotide (D)

Summary: No problems with physical stability encountered

Drug	Dose in syringe (mg)	Volume in syringe (ml)	Concentration (mg/ml)	Diluent	Outcome	Data type
A	400		23.12			
B	1.2	17.3	0.07	Dextrose 5%	Physically stable over 24 h	Laboratory
C	30		1.73			
D	0.3		0.02			

Cyclizine (A), Haloperidol (B), Glycopyrronium (C) and **Octreotide (D)**

Summary: No problems with physical stability encountered. Combination may precipitate as concentrations increase

Drug	Dose in syringe (mg)	Volume in syringe (ml)	Concentration (mg/ml)	Diluent	Outcome	Data type
A	150		7.50			
B	10	20	0.50	Water for injections	Physically stable over 24 h	Clinical observation
C	2.4		0.12			
D	0.6		0.03			

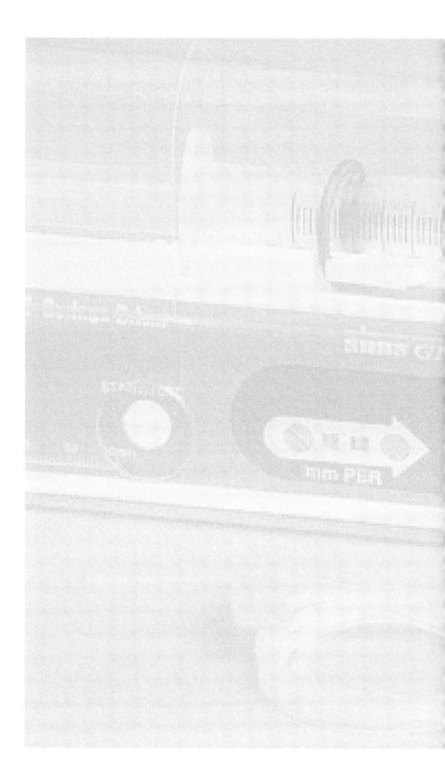

Compatibility data tables

Five drugs

Drug A	B	C	D	E	page
Alfentanil	Cyclizine	Haloperidol	Midazolam	Octreotide	146
Alfentanil	Glycopyrronium	Levomepromazine	Midazolam	Octreotide	146
Diamorphine	Clonazepam	Cyclizine	Dexamethasone	Haloperidol	147
Diamorphine	Cyclizine	Dexamethasone	Haloperidol	Midazolam	147
Diamorphine	Cyclizine	Glycopyrronium	Haloperidol	Midazolam	148
Diamorphine	Cyclizine	Glycopyrronium	Haloperidol	Octreotide	148
Diamorphine	Glycopyrronium	Levomepromazine	Midazolam	Octreotide	149
Diamorphine	Haloperidol	Hyoscine Hydrobromide	Levomepromazine	Midazolam	149
Diamorphine	Hyoscine Butylbromide	Levomepromazine	Midazolam	Octreotide	150

Alfentanil (A), Cyclizine (B), Haloperidol (C), Midazolam (D) and Octreotide (E)

Summary: No problems with physical stability encountered. Combination may precipitate as concentrations increase

Drug	Dose in syringe (mg)	Volume in syringe (ml)	Concentration (mg/ml)	Diluent	Outcome	Data type
A	10		0.53			
B	150		7.89			
C	10	19	0.53	Water for injections	Physically stable over 24 h	Clinical observation
D	20		1.05			
E	0.6		0.03			

Alfentanil (A), Glycopyrronium (B), Levomepromazine (C), Midazolam (D) and Octreotide (E)

Summary: No problems with physical stability encountered. To prevent irritation at the site of infusion, levomepromazine may be given as a subcutaneous injection at doses below 50 mg (= 2 ml)

Drug	Dose in syringe (mg)	Volume in syringe (ml)	Concentration (mg/ml)	Diluent	Outcome	Data type
A	3.5		0.19			
B	2.4		0.13			
C	6.25	18	0.35	Water for injections	Physically stable over 24 h	Clinical observation
D	10		0.56			
E	0.6		0.03			

Diamorphine (A), Clonazepam (B), Cyclizine (C), Dexamethasone (D) and Haloperidol (E)

Summary: No problems with physical stability encountered, although precipitation/turbidity may occur as concentrations increase. Note that a similar rea ction occurs with dexamethasone and haloperidol. Dexamethasone should be given via a bolus subcutaneous injection, or separate CSCI at higher doses

Drug	Dose in syringe (mg)	Volume in syringe (ml)	Concentration (mg/ml)	Diluent	Outcome	Data type
A	50		3.33			
B	2		0.13			
C	150	15	10.00	Water for injections	Physically stable over 24 h	Clinical observation
D	1		0.07			
E	5		0.33			

Diamorphine (A), Cyclizine (B), Dexamethasone (C), Haloperidol (D) and Midazolam (E)

Summary: No problems with physical stability encountered, although precipitation/turbidity may occur as concentrations increase. Note that a similar reaction occurs with dexamethasone and haloperidol. Dexamethasone should be given via a bolus subcutaneous injection, or separate CSCI at higher doses

Drug	Dose in syringe (mg)	Volume in syringe (ml)	Concentration (mg/ml)	Diluent	Outcome	Data type
A	130		15.29			
B	150		17.65			
C	1	8.5	0.12	Water for injections	Physically stable over 24 h	Clinical observation
D	5		0.59			
E	5		0.59			

Diamorphine (A), Cyclizine (B), Glycopyrronium (C), Haloperidol (D) and Midazolam (E)

Summary: No problems with physical stability encountered. Crystallisation may occur as concentrations increase

Drug	Dose in syringe (mg)	Volume in syringe (ml)	Concentration (mg/ml)	Diluent	Outcome	Data type
A	40		2.35			
B	150		8.82			
C	0.8	17	0.05	Water for injections	Physically stable over 24 h	Clinical observation
D	5		0.29			
E	15		0.88			
A	140		6.36			
B	150		6.82			
C	1.6	22	0.07	Water for injections	Physically stable over 24 h	Clinical observation
D	10		0.45			
E	40		1.82			

Diamorphine (A), Cyclizine (B), Glycopyrronium (C), Haloperidol (D) and Octreotide (E)

Summary: No problems with physical stability encountered. Crystallisation may occur as concentrations increase

Drug	Dose in syringe (mg)	Volume in syringe (ml)	Concentration (mg/ml)	Diluent	Outcome	Data type
A	40		2.35			
B	150		8.82			
C	1.8	17	0.11	Water for injections	Physically stable over 24 h	Clinical observation
D	5		0.29			
E	0.6		0.04			

Diamorphine (A), Glycopyrronium (B), Levomepromazine (C), Midazolam (D) and Octreotide (E)

Summary: No problems with physical stability encountered. To reduce irritation at the site of infusion, levomepromazine may be given as a subcutaneous injection at doses below 50 mg (= 2 ml)

Drug	Dose in syringe (mg)	Volume in syringe (ml)	Concentration (mg/ml)	Diluent	Outcome	Data type
A	30		1.25			
B	2.4		0.10			
C	50	24	2.08	Water for injections	Physically stable over 24 h	Clinical observation
D	20		0.83			
E	0.6		0.03			

Diamorphine (A), Haloperidol (B), Hyoscine Hydrobromide (C), Levomepromazine (D) and Midazolam (E)

Summary: No problems with physical stability encountered. To reduce irritation at the site of infusion, levomepromazine may also be given as a subcutaneous injection at doses below 50 mg (= 2 ml)

Drug	Dose in syringe (mg)	Volume in syringe (ml)	Concentration (mg/ml)	Diluent	Outcome	Data type
A	30		1.76			
B	10		0.59			
C	1.2		0.07	Water for injections	Physically stable over 24 h	Clinical observation
D	12.5		0.74			
E	40		2.35			

Diamorphine (A), Hyoscine Butylbromide (B), Levomepromazine (C), Midazolam (D) and Octreotide (E)

Summary: No problems with physical stability encountered. To reduce irritation at the site of infusion, levomepromazine may be given as a subcutaneous injection at doses below 50 mg (= 2 ml)

Drug	Dose in syringe (mg)	Volume in syringe (ml)	Concentration (mg/ml)	Diluent	Outcome	Data type
A	160		9.41			
B	120		7.06			
C	50	17	2.94	Water for injections	Physically stable over 24 h	Clinical observation
D	15		0.88			
E	0.6		0.04			

Appendices

Syringe Driver Prescription

DOCTOR MUST SIGN, DATE AND CLEARLY CROSS THROUGH BOX UPON DISCONTINUATION

Date started	Drug(s) and dose(s)
Date stopped	
Pharmacist	
Doctor's signature	

Date started	Drug(s) and dose(s)
Date stopped	
Pharmacist	
Doctor's signature	

Date started	Drug(s) and dose(s)
Date stopped	
Pharmacist	
Doctor's signature	

Date started	Drug(s) and dose(s)
Date stopped	
Pharmacist	
Doctor's signature	

Date started	Drug(s) and dose(s)
Date stopped	
Pharmacist	
Doctor's signature	

Date started	Drug(s) and dose(s)
Date stopped	
Pharmacist	
Doctor's signature	

Date started	Drug(s) and dose(s)
Date stopped	
Pharmacist	
Doctor's signature	

Date started	Drug(s) and dose(s)
Date stopped	
Pharmacist	
Doctor's signature	

Name: . . . .
Ward: . . . .

Syringe Driver: Nursing Administration Record

All syringe drivers should be checked 4 hourly to ensure site viability, correct delivery and to ensure no crystallization or precipitation has occurred. Nurses should sign below when the driver is started, and every time it is checked. Any problems, such as resiting, should be recorded. Inform the doctor or pharmacist if crystallization or precipitation occurs

Date	Sign	Dose(s)	Time started	0200	0600	1000	1400	1800	2200	Comments

Index